Why Are We Conscious?

Why Are We Conscious?

A Scientist's Take on Consciousness and Extrasensory Perception

David E. H. Jones

Pan Stanford Publishing

Published by

Pan Stanford Publishing Pte. Ltd.
Penthouse Level, Suntec Tower 3
8 Temasek Boulevard
Singapore 038988

Email: editorial@panstanford.com
Web: www.panstanford.com

British Library Cataloguing-in-Publication Data
A catalogue record for this book is available from the British Library.

Why Are We Conscious? A Scientist's Take on Consciousness and Extrasensory Perception

ISBN 978-981-4774-32-1 (Hardcover)
ISBN 978-1-315-16688-9 (eBook)

Printed in Great Britain by Ashford Colour Press Ltd

Contents

Conventions

In this book I condense numbers big and small by means of the 'exponential notation' universal in science. Thus 10^y means '1.0 with the decimal place moved y places to the right' or more simply '1 followed by y noughts'. 10^0 is just 1. 10^{-y} means '1 divided by 10^y, or '1.0 with the decimal point moved y places to the left'. Some scientific numbers are 'pure' (such as the pure number Greek 'pi'; π is 3.14159... but never terminates), but most have a 'dimension'. These are usually made up of 3 common units, the metre (m, slightly more than a yard), the kilogram (kg, about 2.2 pounds) and the second (s), the common unit of time. I put a space between a number and its unit or dimension (e.g. a length of one metre is 1 m). A calculation in MKS dimensions gives its result in MKS. Conveniently, this is generally in the accepted MKS units for that result.

A few further examples may help. Thus the unit of area, a square meter in the MKS system, has the dimension m^2. Where a unit has more than one type of dimension, I join them by a dot or dots. Thus the unit of velocity, metres per second, has the total dimension $m{\cdot}s^{-1}$. The speed of light, c, is very nearly 3.00×10^8 $m{\cdot}s^{-1}$. A non-MKS unit is sometimes more readily comprehensible: thus a big volume is often more understandable as so many cubic kilometers. To use such a volume in a calculation, however, we have to convert it back to MKS units. This is usually easy: in this case 1 km = 10^3 m, so 1 km^3 = 10^9 m^3.

I often refer to very big numbers. A million is 10^6; a billion is 10^9; a trillion is a million million, or 10^{12}. I also often refer to temperature. The Earth is warm—a typical atmospheric temperature might be 290 K, where K is 'degrees Kelvin' or 'degrees Absolute'. Water freezes to ice at nearly 273 K. Absolute zero, which is as cold as you can ever get, is 0 K. The cosmic microwave background which permeates the whole universe, is at about 3 K.

1

The Human Experience

We live in two worlds. The first and most obvious is the public world we all know. It contains the earth with its objects and animals, and the atmosphere and the heavens. We can generally agree on the things in it. In recent centuries a public science of this world has grown up. Anyone can make an observation, perform an experiment, set out a chain of reasoning, and publish the finding for others to examine or challenge. Many events in the physical world are repeatable and publishable; even those which are essentially unpredictable (e.g. nuclear decay in a radioactive atom) often obey publishable statistical laws. Such publications are typically made by specialized scientists, and few people deny the scientific view of the physical world that they have built up.

The second world is private, and inside our own head. Each of us is born, typically lives for a few decades, and then dies. In that time, each of us has private experiences, such as communicating with other beings or adopting a religious faith. Crucially, we are conscious: indeed, this is

Why Are We Conscious? A Scientist's Take on Consciousness and Extrasensory Perception
David E. H. Jones

ISBN 978-981-4774-32-1 (Hardcover), 978-1-315-16688-9 (eBook)
www.panstanford.com

the only thing we directly know. We do not merely react to our surroundings; we are aware of them. This private world may sometimes include very odd single experiences which seem neither predictable nor subject to statistical analysis. Examples include the sudden awarenesses of telepathy, and the sudden birth of a new idea.

The two worlds seldom talk with each other. Indeed, many of those who support the public, scientific sense of the world dismiss the private world as full of nonsense. Numerous strange 'paranormal' or 'psychic' half-beliefs belong there, as do spirits, ghosts, angels, devils and religious beings in general. Many skeptical physical scientists simply discard the whole lot of them as so much hallucination and superstition. This is the dismissive attitude adopted by CSICOP (the Committee for Scientific Investigation of Claims of the Paranormal, later shortened to CSI, the Committee for Skeptical Inquiry).

This book, however, attempts to see whether the two worlds can be combined, at least partly. I have spent most of my working life as a physical scientist, in fact as a chemist, extending that public scientific world. Yet I have grown to respect the private mental world. Where the two worlds collide, science is often feeble and unsatisfying. It has nothing to say about the way that everyone is conscious and self-aware, and that many people see ghosts, communicate with spiritual entities, have psychic experiences, believe in a life before birth or after death, and so on. I feel that it worth imagining what extensions to existing physical science might have to be made for some of these notions to become acceptable. I have mused before on the way we all have an 'unconscious mind', which occasionally pushes stuff 'upstairs' to the conscious mind (Jones[21]). The process often includes a massive distortion, which helps to explain why many 'paranormal' experiences seem not to make sense. I suspect that the unconscious mind sometimes makes contact with an unknown world 'outside our diving bell', a phrase which I use many times in this book. It was originated by the luckless Monsieur Bauby (Bauby[3] and below). That unknown world may contain much information never accessed by physical science. I am reminded that Shakespeare was unsatisfied by many philosophies. In *Hamlet* he denounces Horatio: 'There are more things in heaven and earth, Horatio, than are dreamt of in your philosophy.' Sadly, Horatio never gave his philosophy, but I present a possible one here.

Existing physical science contains several huge puzzles. One of them is consciousness. There is no theory of it at all: physical science says that everything is made of atoms, and nothing made of atoms should be conscious. Charles Sherrington said of consciousness, 'The problem remains where Aristotle left it 2000 years ago'; the philosopher Descartes recognized it but failed to solve it (Chapter 3); the modern philosopher David Chalmers calls it 'the hard problem'—which it is. There is not even a test for consciousness—thus the question 'Is a beetle conscious?' cannot be answered. One simple but trivial way out would simply be to add consciousness to the set of material properties accepted by physical science: length, mass, electric charge and so on. This simply puts the puzzle in a new form: why, among all material objects, do only human beings and some species of higher animal seem to be conscious? This book does not solve the problem, but adds a new notion. I claim that for an object to be conscious, it needs an unconscious mind. This fits the biological suggestion that the higher animals, as well as human beings, have unconscious minds. The unconscious mind was invented and developed almost entirely by psychiatrists, but we all become aware of it when we get a new idea that 'suddenly just pops up' from it (Jones[21]). The unconscious mind is, in my view, one of the most important hypotheses of the 1900s. I suspect that the strong form of artificial intelligence, which claims that a computer might be conscious, has so far failed because nobody has made a computer with an unconscious mind, or has even thought of how to do it. Indeed, consciousness may be the biggest unsolved problem we know about. It seems to occur in the human brain, and in the brains of higher animals; yet brain physiologists have looked in vain for any details that might help them. I glance at some of the technical problems in Chapter 16.

In this book, I explore the idea that the unconscious mind somehow makes contact with an unknown world 'outside our diving bell'. Almost all of us have absorbed the idea that the observable world is not all that there is. Radio, TV, and much computer technology exploits an 'electromagnetic world' which we cannot feel, but which carries information for us. My proposed additional 'unknown world' also fills space and carries information. It may be as physical and simple as the electromagnetic world, but may also have unique properties. Chapter 7 explores the properties it must have to fit into the physical scientific world we know about. If it exists, and occupies the same space as the physical world, it is only weakly coupled to it. In Chapters 16 and 17 I guess at the sort of technical advances which might allow it to be found and, maybe, explored instrumentally—thus it might be observed by a major development in artificial intelligence! My guess is that this world 'outside our diving bell' is the source of the information which is sometimes picked up by the unconscious mind. It may also have inhabitants (like the physical world). Current science has not looked for it, nor stumbled over aspects of it experimentally. This is not surprising: existing scientific instruments have almost all been invented and developed to study the physical world. I surmise that that 'unknown world outside our diving bell' exists and is often partly accessible to the unconscious mind. It may be detectable by novel scientific experiments. My musings here are not unusual. Several other scientists have also sought to explain physical puzzles by proposing unobserved entities and even unobserved universes (I mention Hugh Everett III and his 'many worlds' theory of quantum mechanics in Appendix D). Much of my observational evidence (largely presented in Chapters 8 to 11) comes from the somewhat disreputable field of 'parapsychology'. I need what it can give me, even though it often makes me as a physical scientist feel rather grubby. For the most part it consists of honest human reports; it would be scientific cowardice to ignore them, even when they do not seem to make sense to me.

The sad story of Monsieur Jean-Dominique Bauby concerns the terrible fate he suffered in 1995. A major stroke deprived him of almost all bodily movement. He could only move his left eye. He managed to write a book about his fate—by blinking that eye to a set of alphabetic cards held up by a publisher's assistant. *The Diving Bell and the Butterfly*[3] was a literary account of his tragedy. It invited the reader to imagine a butterfly trapped inside a diving bell. It was very successful, and was even made into a film.

My suspicion is that intellectually, we are in the same sort of predicament today. We know a great deal about the physical world, and scientific observations are steadily telling us more. On the other hand, we know essentially nothing about the possible world outside our physical diving bell. Many scientists deny that there is anything outside it. In Victorian times our understanding of the physical world was so good that physics was thought to be essentially complete. Numerous people these days have the same sort of sense. This book disputes such a view; I reckon we know very little about anything that matters.

One of my reasons is entirely social. Religious views of the world seem emotionally very strong. It impresses me that when a materialist political system collapses (and I am thinking here of the Soviet Union in the 1990s) a lot of popular religious feeling resurfaces. I suspect it was there all the time. The current materialistic Chinese dictatorship fights a steady battle against religious cults. It successfully opposed the Falung Gong religious movement. It dispatched many adherents to labour camps and psychiatric wards to 'cure' their sectarian obsession. But despite such authoritarian antagonism, cults continue to appeal.

In some way we would all like a comforting religious creed to believe in. Few human minds are satisfied by a scientific and materialistic view of the world, and many people yearn for something beyond it. As a result, many strange beliefs survive, not in the public scientific world, but in the private mental one. This book tries to rescue some of them by a guessed extension of physical science. I sketch our current understanding of the physical world in Chapters 2 and 3, and go on to explore some of the issues raised by that possible unknown world. Thus this book starts fairly conventionally, but goes on to be more speculative.

2

The Physical World

THE PHYSICAL WORLD CONTAINS MANY things which scientists have discovered. A book by the two Morrisons, *Powers of Ten*,[29] gives an informative sketch. Here I outline a few scientific findings.

What is the physical world made of?

At present, we reckon that the whole physical world is made of fundamental particles. There are many different kinds (as the physicist Enrico Fermi said, 'If I knew the names of all these particles, I'd be a botanist'). Most are transient, and are seen only in violent particle-collisions. Some may exist as 'exchange particles' holding others together. One worrying claim is that the universe is largely made up of strange stuff called 'dark matter'; it may be particulate, but we know nothing about it. Here I propose to ignore dark matter, and regard the whole universe as being made up of atoms. They consist of three kinds of stable and enduring particle: the proton, the neutron and

Why Are We Conscious? A Scientist's Take on Consciousness and Extrasensory Perception
David E. H. Jones

ISBN 978-981-4774-32-1 (Hardcover), 978-1-315-16688-9 (eBook)
www.panstanford.com

the electron. The proton carries a single positive electric charge of a bit more than 10^{-19} coulombs. The neutron has about the same size and mass as the proton, but is neutral. The electron is about 10^{-30} kg in weight, and is thus much lighter than the other two. It has a negative electric charge equal and opposite to the positive one of the proton. Everything we know about is made up of these three particles, which combine as atoms.

Each atom has a tiny central 'nucleus' which is a tiny assembly of protons and neutrons, like 'a fly in a cathedral'. It accounts for almost all the weight of the atom, but almost none of its size. Around the tiny nucleus fly orbiting electrons, enough to make the atom as a whole electrically neutral. Appendix C discusses the strange quantum-mechanical laws which seem to govern them; it makes sense to regard the electrons as shells of wavelike 'electron density'. Accordingly, an atom does not have a sharp edge; it just fades away. The best we can do is to say that it is about 10^{-10} m across. One atom can combine chemically with another; the two can form a clump or diatomic molecule by an interaction of their outer electron-shells. Further atoms can then add to the clump; many different sorts of such multi-atom 'chemical molecules' are known. Each forms a specific material, such as salt or water. A living object (a virus or a cell, say) is a little structure assembled from many chemical materials. Each part of such a structure probably contains trillions of chemical molecules.

Some atomic nuclei are 'radioactive', i.e. unstable. They last for a while (which can be under a microsecond or over a million years), but ultimately decay unpredictably, releasing energy. The Earth is hot inside, because of present and past radioactive decays within it. This unpredictable decay is, quantum mechanically, an 'uncaused event'. Schmidt[32] has shown that radioactive decay can be predicted a little better than chance by a few rare and gifted people—this is part of the evidence for my feeling that that there is an unknown world outside the diving bell we know about (Chapter 8).

There are a few hundred stable non-radioactive atomic nuclei. Made into atoms by the electron density around them, and often combined further into chemical substances, they make up the whole material world we know about. It is a common claim that the universe is largely made up, not of atomic matter at all, but of 'dark matter' and 'dark energy'. This book, however, takes all matter to be atomic.

Astronomy

Atoms are very small compared to common material objects. Thus there are about 10^{28} atoms in a man. The Earth is made of many more atoms (about 10^{50}) and the Sun of even more (about 10^{60}). The Sun is so hot that astronomers reckon that most of its atoms are almost permanently torn apart by the intensity of its energy. It consists of atomic nuclei surrounded by a swirling mass of electron density, with no nucleus able to hold onto its electrons for any length of time. Nonetheless, the Sun is electrically neutral, and it makes sense to talk of its composition. It is mainly hydrogen and helium, with small amounts of heavier elements. In the hot Sun these are essentially just atomic nuclei surrounded by a twirl of electrons, but if you could extract a bit of Sun-stuff and cool it down, atoms should condense out of it. The Sun is hot because the atomic nuclei in it occasionally collide, and react to heavier elements. Such nuclear reactions generally give out a vast amount of energy. This usually gives the product particles a very high velocity—i.e. makes them extremely hot. Our own current energy crisis has stimulated attempts to imitate the process on Earth.

The Earth is one of 10 planets that go round the Sun in the solar system. Each is kept in its orbit by the pull of gravity. The Earth is about 1.5×10^{11} m from the Sun, and goes round it in an almost circular orbit once a year. The Sun seems a typical star, 1.4×10^{9} m across, but we do not know if planets are a common feature of stars. Our galaxy consists of a cluster of a few hundred billion stars. They are very widely spread: each is about 10^{17} m from its nearest neighbour, perhaps 10^{9} stellar diameters. The galaxy as a whole (whose edge we see in the sky as the Milky Way) is about 10^{21} m across, and has a volume of about 10^{63} m^3. Between its stars is an 'interstellar gas', which in this book I take to be mainly hydrogen atoms, say a million per m^3. Thus it is much more tenuous than a good earthly vacuum (ordinary air contains over 10^{25} molecules per m^3. It is mainly molecular doublets of nitrogen atoms and oxygen atoms.) Interstellar material sometimes also includes highly dilute chemical molecules, and highly dilute dust.

Our galaxy of a few hundred billion stars is not alone. It is one of many. Like ours, each is a cluster of stars, and there are many types. Ours seems to be a spiral galaxy, of which there are lots of other examples. The visible universe has about 10^{11} galaxies, each about 4×10^{22} m from its neighbours. They tend not to be spread evenly, but to be clustered. The space between them seems to be an almost completely empty vacuum. Intergalactic space has, perhaps, only about 100 hydrogen atoms in every cubic metre, much less than the interstellar gas within a galaxy. The galaxies seem to be receding from us, and from each other (this is 'the expansion of the universe'). The rate of expansion is defined by the Hubble constant, for which a good modern value may be about 1 m$\cdot$s^{-1} per 4.2×10^{17} m of distance. Accordingly galaxies more than about 10^{26} m away from us are receding faster than the speed of light, and we can never observe them. Furthermore, in looking far into space we are also looking back in time; the finite speed of light means that we see things not as they are, but as they were when the light was emitted. The furthest objects we can hope to see will have generated that light just after the universe became transparent. This also limits our vision to about 10^{26} m. Accordingly, the volume of space that we are concerned with is a mere 10^{79} m^3, or 10^{70} km^3.

At least one big question remains: what is the whole thing for? Some cosmologists support the Anthropic Principle, in which the entire structure, and the laws which underlie it, exist to make intelligent life possible. I discuss it briefly and unsympathetically in Appendix E.

Many cosmologists also discard the Principle, and have compared it to the trivial proposition that the whole universe was created to produce some other rare phenomenon. Instead of intelligent life, they say, how about ferromagnetism or radioactivity? It distresses me, and many others, that the arrangement revealed by modern science does not seem to have any sort of design or purpose. As the physical theorist Steven Weinberg once said, 'The more the universe seems comprehensible, the more it also seems pointless.' As human beings, we all have a desire for some believable world-story. The old religious ones described the earth as all there was. Heaven was above it and hell beneath it, and God and the Devil played out a drama for the souls of the earthly humans. This was an exciting story; the Anthropic Principle does not, I fear, make a good emotional substitute.

The universe we observe may be only one of many (Appendix C). Accordingly, the notion of an unknown world 'outside our diving bell', with which the human unconscious mind seems able occasionally to make contact, seems worth exploring. In Chapters 16 and 17 I muse on the experimental advances which might lead to a physical instrument that could also do it.

The electromagnetic spectrum

Apart from matter, what else do we find in the physical universe? One of the answers is radiation. The whole saga of the electromagnetic spectrum started with a tiny chunk of it, the visible light seen by our eyes. The eye is our chief sensory organ, and its mighty extensions the telescope, the microscope and the camera have dominated the building of our scientific picture of the world. It was the great Newton who showed that visible light consists of a few colours, from red to violet (summed they make white). Newton did not know that visible light is itself a tiny region of a huge range of radiations. But since his time later scientists have extended visible light into a whole new vast spectrum. Our imperfect mastery of that spectrum is almost a new sense in itself. A good way of classifying those radiations is by frequency. Right down at the low frequencies we have current electricity, which goes better through metal wires than through space. It ranges from the zero frequency d.c. made by batteries, the 50 or so cycles a second of the a.c. that generating stations deliver to our buildings, and the few kilocycles a second handled by sound amplifiers and loudspeakers. Frequencies greater than zero can travel through space. Thus we find radio waves from a few kilocycles a second to many megacycles a second. At higher frequencies we have microwaves, infrared radiation and (at a few hundred trillion cycles a second) visible light. At even higher frequencies come ultraviolet light, X-rays, and gamma rays.

Generally speaking, our technical skill with this spectrum decreases with frequency. At the low end, we can make electricity more or less to order and can accomplish a vast amount with it (the portable electric meters by which we measure voltage, current, frequency, electrical resistance and so on, are practically new senses in themselves). Our skill in generating specific frequencies, and measuring and using them, extends through much of radio, but begins to falter in the microwave region. With infrared radiation, visible light and higher frequencies, we can usually measure a given frequency but have trouble generating it. The goodness of Mother Nature lets us generate a few specific sharp wavelengths (in masers and lasers), but we usually cannot tune around them to play with other wavelengths and frequencies nearby. Astronomy depends on detecting radiation from the sky very sensitively. It has done wonders with visible light, and radio astronomy is advancing rapidly. But much may still remain to be revealed about the universe in the infrared and ultraviolet bands, and even more when we are able to detect and make images from specific frequencies of light and other optical radiations. However, at present our photographic film and photosensitive diodes respond to quite broad ranges of radiation.

Quantum mechanics complicates our understanding of radiation. Newton thought it was a stream of particles, Victorian physicists thought it was waves; quantum mechanics asserts that it is both. Modern physicists reckon that all radiation consists of 'photons', which are particles with a wavelength, but no inherent mass. They all travel through space at the same velocity, that of light—nearly 3.00×10^8 $m \cdot s^{-1}$. (This view fits the theory of quantum mechanics, which I discuss in Appendix C.)

The creation and duration of the universe

Both matter and radiation exist in physical space. The idea once seemed simple: scientists and engineers assumed that there are three dimensions of space, through which we can move freely, and one dimension of time, through which we move steadily and unalterably. (I recall Kipling's powerful phrase, 'the unforgiving minute'.) Recently, scientific space has got more complicated. Fred Hoyle's theory of 'continuous creation' had hydrogen atoms appearing spontaneously in it. There is also a theory that particle-antiparticle pairs can appear briefly in it; this plays a part in the theory of black holes. Some theoretical physicists want more spatial dimensions; I discuss dimensionality in Chapter 7. Nobody seems to have complicated time this way.

Both space and time seem to be infinite, in the sense that you cannot easily imagine an 'edge' to either. When I worked for the Yorkshire Television Company on the science show *Don't Ask Me*, we often got the question from viewers 'Where does space end?'. Since this cannot be answered at all, and certainly not by an entertaining demonstration in a television studio, we ignored it. Time is equally puzzling. The physical laws as we understand them work both forwards and backwards in time; the only one which appears to define a time direction is the second law of thermodynamics. It asserts that entropy (a measure of randomness) always increases, so that the temperature differences of the world (a mark of non-randomness) must on average always decrease. This implies that the universe began with an extremely small entropy. Theories exist in which both space and time are closed but circular, so that (like the surface of the Earth) you never come to an edge but there is only a certain amount of them. Such ideas have an appeal, but they do not amount to a theory. If space is indeed curved enough to close up on itself, a powerful enough telescope would show you the back of your own head.

Space is strange stuff. It exists to hold material—that is why the notion was invented. But it has other abilities too. The fact that light can be transmitted through it used to worry physicists. They invented a 'luminiferous ether' filling all space, through which light could travel (as sound does through air). Then the great physicist James Maxwell considered the strange fact that electric fields and magnetic fields can go through space as well, seemingly without an ether to transmit them (although some physicists invented ethers for these too). He showed that electric and magnetic forces should generate 'electromagnetic radiation', and calculated that it travelled at the speed of light. Physicists soon decided that light was simply Maxwell's theoretical electromagnetic radiation and began to explore other regions of the electromagnetic spectrum.

Space does not merely hold matter and transmit radiation. It transmits forces, usually classified as 'fields', such as those of electricity, magnetism, and gravity. This is a form of 'action at a distance'. Newton accepted it but declined to propose any hypothesis to account for it. Faraday not only accepted it, he invented the 'lines of force' by which the force exerted by a field at any distance can be assessed and calculated. Physicists nowadays tend to dislike it and avoid it. Thus of the four forces whose explanation previously required fields acting at a distance, three are now felt to work by the exchange of particles. Thus, roughly speaking, the strong nuclear force is now thought to be caused through an exchange of gluons; the weak nuclear force is due to the exchange of bosons; the electric and magnetic forces occur by the exchange of photons. Gravity is still an exception, and does not fit this picture. A particle, the 'graviton' has been invented for it, but nobody has seen one or devised an experiment to support its existence. Einstein explained gravity as due to the bending of space-time. If gravity could also be explained by particle exchange, the proposed Theory of Everything would come a step closer.

The scale of space and time

A very powerful modern question, an important advance over the questions asked by the ancient Greek philosophers, concerns time. How old is our universe? And how did it come about? Before about 1600, most writers reckoned that the world has always been much as we see it now. It consisted mainly of the Earth, and was created only a few thousand years ago. In the 1700s, geologists began to challenge this view. They took the present Earth as the result of many changes over time (for example, alterations of sea level). Their theories implied a lot of past time. The Darwinian evolution of life, first promulgated in 1859, took the bold step of applying this philosophy to the origin of plant and animal species. Evolution required many millions of years. Modern cosmology applies it to the whole universe, and requires even more time. One of the questions it asks is, How did the present structure of galaxies and stars arise? The current theory is that it all started with the Big Bang. One of the key pieces of evidence for this is the weak 'cosmic microwave background' which seems to fill all space. It was discovered accidentally in the 1960s, by workers at the Bell Telephone Company who were investigating the sky microwave background against which a communication satellite would have to operate. Russian scientists have called this background 'relic radiation'. They argue that the Big Bang created a huge blast of radiation, and the subsequent expansion of the universe has greatly lengthened its wavelength. The recession of the galaxies lets us date the Big Bang roughly by calculating the time when that expansion began. It comes out as about 13 billion years ago. Similarly, our feelings for the future must now extend into a comparable temporal remoteness.

Nobody has any good theory of how or why creation happened. Current physical theory allows a vacuum to generate a single particle and its anti-particle out of nothing: but the spontaneous creation of a whole universe out of nothing seems to push the idea far beyond anything feasible. An even stranger idea is that the matter and anti–matter thus created may be very slightly different, so that their subsequent mutual annihilation would leave the universe of matter which we observe. This notion says nothing about the so-called dark matter, which some theorists reckon is the major component of the universe, but of which nothing is known. But even if there was any believable theory of creation, deeper questions remain. How did space and time themselves come into existence? And why are there three dimensions of space and one of time? There seems not to be any logical or scientific answer. My notion of a non-physical world, outside our 'diving bell' but fitting into it, adds to the problem but does not suggest any solution to it.

Apart from matter and radiation, what else may be in the physical world? One answer is 'information', which at its most general is the non-uniform distribution of matter and radiation. Thus matter can be organized into the non-uniform distribution which is print; radiation can be organized into the non-uniform distribution which is a radio or television transmission. I discuss living things, and the information in them, in Chapter 3.

3

Life and Its Information

NOBODY KNOWS HOW LIFE WORKS. Neither physicists nor chemists have ever been able to make a living object from non-living matter. Up to about the 1700s it might have been possible to claim, for example, that flies were naturally generated in dung. But careful study disproved such claims, and it is now admitted that the 'spontaneous generation' of life never happens. Life can only arise from seeds created by previous life.

The theory of evolution, initiated by Charles Darwin in the 1800s and developed by innumerable biologists since, envisages life beginning, somehow, as single microscopic 'cells' a few billion years ago. Many single-celled microscopic organisms (such as bacteria) still flourish, but the creatures we are familiar with consist of lots of cells clumped together. Each grew by the steady multiplication of one original cell, often created by a process of sexual reproduction.

A cell is a little closed container, maybe about 0.1 mm across. Inside it is a subtle aqueous paste which

Why Are We Conscious? A Scientist's Take on Consciousness and Extrasensory Perception
David E. H. Jones

ISBN 978-981-4774-32-1 (Hardcover), 978-1-315-16688-9 (eBook)
www.panstanford.com

biologists often call 'protoplasm' and which, among many other things, carries the information that defines the cell. It grows, and the cell expands, till it reaches some critical size; then the cell splits into two cells, which in multicellular organisms stick together. The information it carries divides as well, so that its two 'daughter' cells have it too. This process goes on until, in growing up, a mature multicellular organism may have trillions of cells. Furthermore, not all that information gets expressed. In a human being, for example, some growing cells turn into brain cells, some become stomach or liver cells, and so on. Yet every cell seems to have enough information in it to define the whole body.

A feasible biochemical mechanism for all this was worked out in the 1950s by James Watson and Francis Crick. They proposed that each cell carried its genetic information as sets of long paired molecules, twined together into the famous 'double helix' of DNA (desoxyribonucleic acid). The two intertwined chains of the DNA helix were composed basically of a long sequence of four 'organic base' units. During cell division, each chain molecule unwound into two single chains, one of which went into each new daughter cell. These were completed in the two daughters by a molecular reconstruction, turning each long molecule into a double helix again.

Reproduction is another informational puzzle. Why do acorns grow into oak trees, lions beget more lions, and human beings have human babies? This too was fitted into the DNA theory. Biologists had already reckoned that each cell has a certain number of genetic chemical entities called 'genes', coupled into objects (sometimes visible under the microscope) called 'chromosomes'. In the process of sexual reproduction, two special cells fuse into one. This by itself would give the newly fertilized egg too much information, but the process 'throws out' half the chromosomes randomly. The new cell then has the right number of chromosomes to go on living, and to grow up into a new individual. That discard also makes each generation vary; a new baby is related to its parents but is not identical to either. Watson and Crick identified the chromosomes as long helical chains of the same double helices of DNA by which they explained cell division. In human beings, each cell has 22 such helices, plus one pair of the 'autosome chains', which determine sex. Hence each cell carries its genetic information as 46 molecular entities in all. A typical chromosome may contain about 2000 genes (certain chromosomes have about 4500 genes; others only about 500). The whole assembly of genes in the chromosomes makes up the 'genome' or 'genetic code' of that human being.

The DNA theory does not explain how organisms acquire information in the first place, nor how they come to know some things instinctively. Thus a baby bird knows the song appropriate to its species, although it has not learnt it. It is coded somehow in its DNA. One geneticist has remarked that it cannot be a succession of 'note' symbols in that DNA, or the occasional bird would sing its song backwards. Similarly, human children seem to inherit from their parents the 'need' to acquire language, but no sort of vocabulary or grammar. A historical experiment, which we should now denounce as very cruel, had children not brought up to speak any language. The idea was to find out what language they would speak naturally. One favourite guess was that they would speak Hebrew, this being God's language. Modern experience, in which adults speaking mutually incomprehensible languages have raised children, have found that these children invent a linguistic 'creole' by which they can talk amongst themselves. It interests me that it takes many years to learn any language, whether a private creole or a mature one spoken by adults. This may reflect the slow maturation of our nervous and mental equipment. Chapter 7 notes that our memory is still very immature at birth, which raises questions about what memories we may retain of life in the womb.

All living things die in the end and are eaten: either by the predator that killed them, or by other predators, or by (for example) fungi or bacteria. What happens to the information in the body chemicals? Being specific to the body that carried it, it is dangerous to the eater. It is coded in the way in which the coupled bases are linked in the DNA of that body, and in the linked chains of amino acids—proteins—that the DNA has created. Digestion destroys this information by breaking the food down, largely into an alphabet of single bases and single amino acids. The resulting 'soup' then ceases to be carry information or be dangerous to the eater, and may be used by it to build structures carrying its own information.

My rather old natural history books tend to ignore such internal chemistry. Their ideal reader, I feel, would be examining a dead specimen. Many geologists classify and date rocks by the fossils they find in them: shells and bones and suchlike (very tiny creatures in the rock might require a microscope). The type and abundance of the extant creatures changes greatly over time—which is itself evidence that evolution has occurred. My books give a lot of detail about e.g. the skeleton of a specimen, the number and the nature of its teeth, and what other species it might have been related to. And indeed, biology advances by amassing huge numbers of such physical details. As with all science, it is ultimately based on careful observations, and not at all on the state of mind of whoever made those observations. It is largely by studying such observations that Darwin built the evidence to buttress his mighty theory of evolution. This asserts that while species seem immutable in the short term (so that, for example, lions always beget more lions) they can vary in the long term—which Darwin felt was many millions of years. His argument, supported by many biological facts, was that each act of sexual reproduction gave offspring which varied slightly. The variations which improved the species had a better chance of surviving and having offspring in their turn (the so-called survival of the fittest). So the species slowly changed. On a long enough time scale, all living things may have evolved from just one ancestor.

A feature of evolution theory that greatly annoyed its first hearers was its implication that human beings evolved from animals, and indeed that man is an animal himself. That is why he has the same sort of ground plan as many animals, and the same sort of sensory equipment (eyes, ears, and so on). Those senses have the same purpose too: to observe the physical world, and make biologically useful deductions about it. Thus a predator such as a lion makes a characteristic noise or set of noises, apparent to the ears. It has a characteristic shape and way of moving, apparent to the eyes. It has a characteristic smell, apparent to the nose. It can leave footprints, again apparent to the eyes. The brain can interpret all this sensory data and think, 'Lion! Over there! Beware!'

Is the brain just a digital computer?

One almost automatic technical musing is that the brain of a man or of a higher animal is simply a computer. Indeed, many thinkers have imagined that an animal, and even a human being, is just a robot driven by a computing brain. This theory pictures one of these higher creatures as a body, a brain, and two sets of nerves connecting them. The sensory set of nerves has the job of transmitting data to the brain. Thus a nerve ending in the skin may send a message to the brain about the pressure it is feeling; one in the retina of an eye will transmit data about part of the image which that eye is viewing. The brain then considers all this sensory information. Many living organisms, including us, give the impression of having a specific set of goals, such as the desire to survive and the desire to reproduce. In this robotic theory, the brain runs the body so as to maximize the likelihood of achieving those goals. When it has worked out the best way of exploiting current condition so as to achieve them, it activates its decision. It sends orders to another set of 'motor nerves' which go from the brain to various muscles in the body. The body then executes the actions which the brain has determined.

Thus the whole organism is simply an elaborate robot. Since it is just a machine, there is no need to tackle the 'hard problem' of why it is conscious–if it is. And indeed it may be. The strong form of artificial intelligence asserts, in one of its forms, that consciousness is simply a by-product of handling information. Any sufficiently complex device for processing information will become conscious of the information it is processing. If an animal brain meets those so-far-undetermined criteria, it will be conscious too.

At present, nobody understands those criteria, if indeed they exist. Nobody has made a computer that even seems conscious, nor has anyone made a believable quasi-human robot guided by a computer 'brain'. Yet these ideas retain their appeal: designers are making the effort. Humanlike robots have even been given the name 'androids'. 'Marvin, the paranoid android', is an amusing fictional robot in Douglas Adams's *The Hitchhiker's Guide to the Galaxy*. Google has a computer operating system called Android.

Thus the whole idea of an animal or a human being as a conscious robot makes a neat theory, but I do not believe it at all. My feeling is that no atomic system, even one given senses and organized into a system driven by a digital computer, can be conscious in this way. Nonetheless, the proposition makes sense and deserves discussion.

Human beings and the higher animals rather give the impression of being physical robots driven by a central computer, so why are they conscious? The philosopher Descartes raised the problem of animal consciousness over 300 years ago and was unable to answer it convincingly. In about 1640 he imagined a world of 'matter in motion' entirely made up of material particles hitting each other. This picture fitted the physical science of the time. He could not imagine any way in which a conscious entity could arise in such a world. He found himself driven to invent a human 'soul' somewhere in the brain. His guess located it in the pineal gland—at the time, this gland was thought not to exist in animal brains. The soul, he said, has the job of translating the physical information conveyed by our senses into the conscious mental constructs that inform the mind. It also performs the reverse job—taking conscious mental constructions such as intentions, and converting them into commands for our muscles. He saw this physical-mental dualism, as operated by the pineal gland, to be uniquely human. He was happy to regard even the higher animals as mere unconscious automata, and rejected the whole concept of cruelty to animals. He once threw a cat off a roof to demonstrate his belief that it was simply an automatic machine. He had more trouble in squaring his notions of the human soul with the ones expounded by the Roman Catholic Church (one critic said of him that 'he threw cats well, but Popes badly').

Over 300 years after Descartes, we still do not understand consciousness. Alan Turing's famous paper[35] 'Can a Machine Think?' touches on the problem, but does not solve it. It imagines a judge faced by two teleprinters, one of which goes to a human being, and the other to a machine. The judge can type anything he wants on either of the teleprinters, so as to receive its reply or maintain a printed conversation. If the judge cannot tell which teleprinter goes to the human being and which to the machine, then you have made a machine that can think. The paper mentions telepathy (Chapter 8) and other aspects of extrasensory perception as a power which the human mind might be able to deploy, while no machine can deploy it. It mentions the common cliché that a human being is conscious because it has a piece of apparatus called a 'soul'. Descartes, like me, must have been baffled by the idea that a soul could make a human body conscious. Turing seems to reckon that the idea has enough coherence to deserve mention, though he does not discuss consciousness in animals. We seem generally to assume that an animal does not have a soul, but it can have an equivalent 'anima'—an entity that does not survive death, though a soul does. What happens to the soul when it leaves the body at death is expounded by various religious dogmas. (The Victorian poet Cosmo Monkhouse has a moving poem, 'Any Soul to Any Body', in which he imagines the soul grieving over the loss of the body. I also recall a story for children, whose characters are children themselves. They observe their Nanny bringing them food, dressing them, and so on, but ponder that she may be doing all this as a mere stock, an unconscious thing, because her soul has been stolen by dwarves.)

We still do not understand how any material object, such as an animal or a man, can be conscious. However, a few useful limits have recently been suggested. Thus Marian Dawkins has pointed out that a conscious creature will experience discomfort or pain, only if the sensation reflects a useful signal for avoiding damage. A plant, which has no mechanism for avoiding damage, is unlikely to feel pain; indeed, although plants are clearly living biological objects, nobody imagines that they are conscious. Even so, it is natural to imagine that biology is important for consciousness. The only objects that we feel to be conscious are that small subset of biological objects which have brains. Indeed, we commonly assume that the brain is the seat of consciousness, though some thinkers in artificial intelligence claim that any sufficiently complex information-handling system will become conscious of the information it is handling. So it is natural to look for some clue to material consciousness in the brain.

Brain physiologists, like philosophers, have never explained how a brain can be conscious. Indeed, consciousness puzzles biologists as well. How did it evolve? In what way does a conscious creature have an advantage over one which is not conscious? If they behave the same way, there is no advantage, and consciousness should not have evolved. If they behave differently, you should be able to identify that difference and use it to decide if a creature is conscious. My sense is that consciousness only has value for animals which communicate with each other. Solitary, non-pack animals would gain nothing by being conscious, so they would not evolve consciousness even if it were part of the evolutionary repertoire. Furthermore, if consciousness is an evolutionary product, a conscious creature ought to have that fact somewhere in its DNA code. I have mused on the possibility of finding the DNA code for consciousness. An alternative theory, which appeals to advocates of artificial intelligence, and which I mention above, is that any sufficiently complex information-handling system (such as a human being or a higher animal), automatically becomes conscious of the information it is handling. If this is just how information-handling systems work, understanding it would explain consciousness, and it would have no relevance to the evolutionary process. My theory that to be conscious at all, you need an unconscious mind, seems to imply that the unconscious mind evolved. Creatures with an unconscious mind had a subtle advantage over creatures without one. It came to be exploited in the communications between animals in a pack. This theory is expounded by the biologist Robert Trivers[34]. Human beings have developed the unconscious mind further, in ways which sometimes interest psychiatrists.

In the early part of the 1900s, the brain was often compared to a telephone exchange (which also routes electrical signals through a vast number of switches). These days, our preferred technical analogy is with the digital computer. So it is worth looking at computer technology. Each element of a working digital computer only has two states, off (usually 0 volts) and on (usually a few volts). Its working instructions, and the numbers they work on, are all made up of these discrete digital voltages. Their exact intensities and durations do not matter, though some clock system usually decides if a sustained neuronal pulse of (say) 0 volts, is really several 0s in series. Douglas Hofstadter and Daniel Dennett[11] expound some of the problem of the brain, the computer, and consciousness. Hofstadter takes a strong 'artificial intelligence' position (Chapter 16). He has imagined that a brain might be conscious even if the cells composing it are not. Thus his imaginary 'Aunt Hillary' is an ant heap, conscious although composed of unconscious ants. An English tradition is that, if an important human event like a death occurs in the family, the family beekeeper has to 'tell the bees'. The colony needs to know about its human overseers. Like Hofstadter, I can imagine that a colony of social insects might act as a 'super-organism' and have a collective consciousness, in the same sort of way that a multicellular organism like a man can feel itself to be an individual. It interests me that the bees may not understand spoken English; the colony, perhaps, reacts to conscious thoughts before they get translated into language.

Now the brain is certainly 'digital': indeed, the early computers were known in popular parlance as 'electronic brains'. The brain is digital in the sense that its billions of brain cells (neurons) exchange digital nerve pulses among each other, and that these pulses seem to convey information by their number or frequency, and not (for example) by their intensity or duration. When a brain cell 'fires', it generates a specific electrical output 'pulse', which then travels down all the output nerves of the neuron, mainly to other neurons.

This digital output certainly seems fundamental to how the brain works; if it goes wrong, the patient thinks and behaves in a damaged and non-human way. The brain, like the rest of the body, is liable to invasion by foreign organisms (the immune system is part of our defence mechanism). In addition, it can be sabotaged by internal failures, such as Alzheimer's disease and Huntington's chorea. These terrible diseases seem to prevent part of the brain from working digitally. They create in specific neurons one or more 'neurofibrillary tangles' of protein molecules which destroy the digital effectiveness of that neuron. So far, no treatment has been found to inhibit or reverse the degradation.

There are (at least) three ways in which a brain differs from a computer. Firstly, a computer is very much faster. Secondly, a computer goes in for a lot of coding, while the brain seems not to. Thirdly, a computer is a deterministic device, while the brain seems a typical sloppy, biological, probabilistic one.

Let us consider these in order. It takes about a millisecond for one neuron to send a digital pulse to another; one transistor can send such a pulse to another in about a nanosecond. Accordingly, if there are a hundred thousand million neurons in the brain, a computer with a hundred thousand transistors—which is entirely possible—could conduct as many switching operations every second as a brain does. So, if you only knew how to connect its transistors, you might make a computer that mimicked a brain.

Coding is fundamental to every computer. Not only does it translate any command from a program into an 'internal machine language', but if (for example) its task requires it to multiply two numbers, it has to find and implement the microcode to do it. The basic 'architecture' of the computer, due to John von Neumann, has many such microcodes. At present, computer technologists are considering the advantages of having fewer codes arranged as a 'reduced instruction set'. When a computer, using all those microcodes, has completed a program, it has to conduct a final decoding: that of turning its answer into a form that its human operator will understand. By contrast the brain, while it does have a digital code, has one very simple one. A skin sensor, for example, may have the job of transmitting to the brain the pressure which it is feeling. It makes no attempt to generate a signal whose intensity reflects that pressure. It obeys the 'all or none' code for nerves, such that the smallest pressure of interest corresponds to a single sharp digital pulse. If it feels a higher pressure it will send several sharp pulses, such that their number or rate rises with pressure. At the receiving end, the brain deduces the pressure by adding up the pulses. This simple system makes excellent biological sense; it is almost unaffected by small errors. Suppose the sensor sends 100 pulses. If one pulse is missed or another gets in, the received message is slightly wrong: 99 or 101.

But the brain does not crash or go wild, and its response to the message is nearly correct. Brain physiologists seem not to have found any other codes.

A computer is a deterministic device. It must never make an error—for just one may crash it. By contrast, the brain seems very sloppy. The pulse from a neuron may be received by up to a thousand others, and on its reception it may cause a receiving neuron to fire in its turn. Even so, this may not be certain. Another input pulse, perhaps from another neuron, may make the recipient even more likely to fire. I feel that a brain neuron is too sloppy to be the biological analogue of a deterministic computer element.

Thus, I reject the notion that the brain is just a biological computer. A computer, in essence, is a device made of hardware to run whatever 'software' can be fed into it. Another name for that 'software' is the 'program', which it applies to the data it is given. In every modern computer it is stored. The 'stored program' computer was undoubtedly one of the major inventions of the 1900s. I recall the struggle I had to understand it. Computers these days have both program and data stored in its global memory, in different places but in an identical fashion. A big stored program can be far larger and more complex than the small data set it is given to work on—if this happens often, the perpetrator can be accused of 'number crunching'. Hofstadter felt that a computer might be conscious not from its 'hardware' but from its 'software', its program. In a sense, the hardware is the instrument, but the software is the music. This idea fits the notion that an information-processing system can be conscious, but I have failed to understand it.

Why does biology duck out of precision wherever it can? I once saw an almost biological slogan: a pharmacist's sign proclaiming 'We dispense with accuracy'. Even where biology needs precision, as in the eye (which grows in the embryo in darkness), the outcome is seldom perfect. Maybe half my readers will be viewing these words through correcting glass spectacle lenses. Human technology, including that of computers, greatly exploits precision. In the old days, people such as Chippendale were much admired for making things precise, so that they fitted smoothly and exactly. These days, the rise of precision interchangeable engineering parts has led us all to expect that a new component, no matter where or when it was made, will fit a machine exactly and replace a failed component perfectly. We are used to precision, and expect it almost automatically.

Biology is quite different. Every biological entity must continue to function even if its state is highly imperfect. Among other distresses, it will be under attack from micro-organisms, will carry a load of parasites, may have to live with previously inflicted damage and wounds, and will continue to suffer, in Hamlet's words, 'the thousand natural shocks that flesh is heir to'. Despite all this damage, it still has to go on working. Like all the rest of the organism, the brain must expect and be resilient to such shocks—I discuss below the way it can often survive the massive injury of a stroke. Some physiologists feel that it stores several copies of important data in different places, so that even if one copy is lost, there's a good chance that another will survive.

The brain probably has many other tasks than storing and handing data, and again, that lack of precision ought to help. Thus, among its many routine jobs, the brain probably keeps an eye on the calcium-magnesium ratio of the blood. It would probably not even notice a change of 1 part per million. But if that ratio shifts by (say) 10 percent, the brain might initiate the right biochemistry to bring it back. We all have 'free will', so do many animals, and I reckon that it just arises from our biological sloppiness.

The structure of the brain

To the student, a brain just looks like a lump of grey porridge. Even to the brain surgeon, with great feeling for its many regions and their specific associations with parts of the body, the brain as a whole has a sameness about it. And on the microscale, its seeming planlessness looks very discouraging. It may of course have a fine structure too subtle for the microscopist to discern. It consists of a mass of 'grey matter' (that vast number of neurons or brain cells saluted by, among others, Hercule Poirot). These grey cells are joined by nerves, 'white matter'. A human brain has about 100 billion (10^{11}) grey cells, each about 0.1 mm across and connected to about a thousand others. The connecting white matter 'wires' or 'processes' may be less than 1 mm or more than 1000 mm long. They may branch. At their ends, or at intervals along their length, are little knoblike entities, called 'synapses' each of which makes close contact with another process, or another neuron. It is those synapses which transmit the nervous impulses from one neuron to another.

Useful information about the brain can sometimes be obtained from various forms of brain failure. A stroke, for example (I have had one), causes failure of part of the brain, sometimes by blocking the blood supply to some brain cells, so that they cease to obtain food and oxygen, and sometimes by the breakage of a blood vessel, so that the local brain cells are flooded with blood and cannot operate. In either case, the affected region of brain becomes useless connective tissue. A stroke often disrupts the victim's physical skills—such as those of dexterity, balance or language. This shows that some feature of such skills is indeed held in the brain. However, if the victim is supported over time (as I was) he or she often recovers many elements of those lost skills. Given time, a lot of brain activity seems to be movable from a damaged and useless part of the brain to some different region. This seems to suggest that the brain as a whole is not heavily used, either for storage or processing. Parts of it can often accept new duties. My own stroke seems to have erased much information about the event and its treatment, but I can still recall many old memories. I suspect that the brain may indeed hold the same information in several different places. The original site is generally accessed for that information, but the same data may also be held in a garbled or compressed form in other sites elsewhere. This is why the return of stroke-erased memories and abilities often takes a lot of time. The system has to unscramble and restore the information held in the 'reserve' sites. In my own case, my bank demanded a new copy of my signature, to replace the version that it had on file. My signature seemed not have been changed by that stroke, but I imagine that a bank serving millions of customers will have encountered stroke victims who were able to return to the bank, but with a different signature. This suggests to me that the slow and sometimes partial return of rapidly lost data might give useful clues as to where in the brain that data, both memories and abilities, might be stored. This in turn implies the question: where in the brain is the unconscious mind? If it occupied a specific region of the brain, it should be recognized by anatomists; it seems not to be. Furthermore, expert psychiatrists should occasionally encounter a stroke victim in whom that post-stroke brain reorganization moved a repressed memory out of the unconscious mind and into a region where it was apparent to consciousness. The stroke victim might then become aware of it: it might even have a detectable and beneficial psychiatric effect on him or her. I never saw anything like this either in myself or in any of the other stroke patients in the neurological unit. I have never read of any such event. This supports my suggestion that some part of our unconscious mind may not be held in the brain at all. It might be somewhere else in the body or even outside it entirely—in fact in the unknown world outside our diving bell.

Another way of trying to explore the consciousness of the brain is to study brainy animals which seem to be conscious. As Trivers noted, consciousness seems to occur in pack species; it may feature in interactions such as communication. Some birds (crows and parrots come to my mind) have very small brains but show remarkable skill in understanding a visual scene, reacting to sound, and even making a sound. There has even been parrot who seemed able to maintain a meaningful conversation with a human being. This makes me wonder not merely how a brain can be conscious, but how much information it can acquire and handle. For the human brain, I try to explore this thesis in Appendix D. There I make a very rough estimate of the amount of information that a human brain can store. My feeing is that we can all access more information than this, and that therefore we hold some information outside the brain. Furthermore, I reckon that the human brain is not heavily used anyway: in practice it holds much less than this. If challenged by an event like a stroke, it can shift information around into unused areas. Most physiologists, of course, assume without question that everything we know is held in the brain in material form. I feel free to question this assumption. The calculation of Appendix D is certainly very rough, and open to many sorts of question. Nonetheless, it seems consistent with the suggestion that we know more that the physical brain can hold. This is supported by the idea that the unconscious mind is much bigger than the conscious one—though we know nothing of its size, let alone its contents. I like the idea that some of our memories are held not in the brain but in that unknown world outside our diving bell, 'in the cloud' as computer users sometimes say. This notion seems to me to be a way of escaping the impact of that terrible African saying, 'When a man dies, a library is burned down.'

4

The Unconscious Mind

THIS DISCUSSION OF THE STRUCTURE of the brain implies its main and most mysterious property: it is conscious. Since consciousness is the only thing of which we are directly aware, it is massively important. Indeed in this book I make the bold claim that the unconscious mind is essential for consciousness: to be conscious at all, you need an unconscious mind. The unconscious mind is, in my view, one of the most important hypotheses of the 1900s. No matter what the unconscious mind does, or what information it may hold, or where it may be, it plays a vital role in human life. The unconscious mind may have been first imagined by the great Frederick Myers, who was such a notable early figure in the Society for Psychical Research, but it was greatly developed by the psychiatrists Sigmund Freud and Carl Jung. Most psychologists regard it as existing somewhere in the brain; yet brain anatomists seem not to have identified any region of the brain which might hold it. This allows me to speculate that it may not be in the brain at all; indeed I can even imagine that parts

Why Are We Conscious? A Scientist's Take on Consciousness and Extrasensory Perception
David E. H. Jones

ISBN 978-981-4774-32-1 (Hardcover), 978-1-315-16688-9 (eBook)
www.panstanford.com

of it occupy the non-material world outside our diving bell. That may help to explain why psychiatrists can only get at bits of it. We know nothing about its overall size or content.

Some animals may have unconscious minds: an idea that has been put forward and developed by Trivers[34]. He has suggested that it is inherently deceptive, and holds truths that the conscious mind needs to lie about. I like the idea, and discuss unconscious deceitfulness later in this chapter. Some psychiatrists hold that occasionally a bit of the human unconscious mind gets so far into the conscious mind of an individual as actually to be uttered. When such a damaging contradiction occurs, it is often called a 'Freudian slip'. I have claimed elsewhere[21] that the unconscious human mind is often kept active by playing with the ideas, troubles, and contradictions that get down to it, and that just as the grit in an oyster occasionally creates a pearl, so some the brilliant and novel ideas that sometimes just 'pop up' in the human mind were built there by the unconscious (I mention this claim later in the chapter). The psychiatrist Carl Jung, in his own musings on the unconscious mind, proposed a human 'collective unconscious', which may be an extension of the 'great memory' imagined by the poet William Yeats. Jung proposed that all human beings are joined in some way to a collective unconscious mind. He put the idea forward in about 1916, and seems to have based it on the striking consistency in which certain symbols and images, which he called 'archetypes', occur in folklore, fairy tales, dreams and delusions. This idea supports the notion that all human beings have fairly similar minds, but it seems not to imply any connection between living ones. The idea of a human 'collective unconscious' may be supported by the rare human experience of telepathy (Chapter 8). If one assumes that telepathy is a process conducted by the unconscious mind, which occasionally transmits information to other human beings, then we may indeed all be linked by Jung's collective unconscious. Jung himself seems not to have taken his notion further. Thus I have heard of two people who claim to have had the same dream, but Jung, who often analyzed dreams, seems never to have suggested that the dream of a client came from someone else, and gave insight into that someone else. However, it is possible that the collective unconscious, like human telepathic power and our neglected sense of smell, is a vestigial relic of some former animal ability. Rupert Sheldrake has even proposed that pet animals may communicate telepathically with their human owners (Chapter 8). The collective unconscious also fits my own speculation that some of our mental information is held in non-material form in the unknown world outside our diving bell, and can be sometimes be transmitted to other minds. It can even be somehow stored in that world (Chapter 7) so that it is available to others after the death of the owner.

We are all aware of consciousness in ourselves. We happily attribute it to other human beings, and to many animals. The main point of keeping an animal as a pet is to enjoy its relationship with you as one conscious creature to another. We are less sure about the consciousness of more primitive creatures. Is a frog conscious? A few years ago I would have guessed no; but a paper about the behaviour of male and female tree-frogs, their relationship to each other and to their tadpoles, changed my mind. There is no good test for consciousness; only a feeling about it. We can feel that some creatures (such as a pet animal) are conscious, and some things (such as a hand calculator, despite the speed it imparts one in doing arithmetic calculations) are not. Yet the question has many important aspects. For example, is a beetle conscious? If not, and a beetle is a mere biological machine, it is impossible to be cruel to a beetle. Biologists can devise new and informative experiments which damage beetles, without being worried by ethical concerns.

It puzzles me that only certain living things, all with carbon-based chemistry, are conscious. This apparent dependence on chemistry does not make sense. No system of atoms, whether based on carbon or on any other element, should ever be conscious at all. Furthermore, I feel that there is nothing special about carbon. A conscious entity might be based on silicon, or germanium, or not be based on any particular chemistry. Artificial intelligence, or AI, claims in its strong form that a conscious computer is possible; indeed, one of its notions is that any information-processing system may become conscious of the information it is processing. By contrast, the thesis of this text is that for anything to be conscious, it needs an unconscious mind.

Nobody has a good theory of the unconscious mind. In Chapter 16 I discuss the notion that a computer might be made to have an unconscious mind, but I cannot imagine any useful technical details, and fail to provide any. Indeed, technicians never seem to have discussed what form an unconscious mind might take in a computer, or how one might build a computer that has one. However, I like the idea. If built, it might be able to test, and perhaps disprove, my notions about consciousness.

The 'chattering monkey' theory: does the conscious mind shout down the unconscious one?

Many psychiatrists, and at least one novelist, have speculated that the unconscious mind is much bigger than the conscious mind. And yet we know nothing about it. Freud has proposed that it forms the basis of the true personality. His 'id' lives there, and much psychiatry is devoted to recovering 'repressed memories' or 'repressed aspects of the personality' which are pushed down there, so that the conscious mind can never be aware of them. Occasionally the unconscious mind pushes new and important creative ideas up into the conscious mind, and these sudden mental explosions can sometimes transform their whole field. I have noted several intriguing examples[23] of such sudden creative insights. Yet the unconscious mind is usually quite silent. Since I suspect that the unconscious mind may be crucial for consciousness, I am very interested in the idea that it sometimes tries weakly to touch that consciousness.

One common notion of normal life is that our awareness is dominated by the loud 'chattering monkeys' of the conscious mind. To become aware of the quiet voice of the unconscious mind, we need to 'still' those chattering monkeys. This makes some sort of sense; our mental efforts are usually centred on what the brain is telling us consciously. We are always aware of the inputs to it from our senses, its cogitations on what they imply about the world around us, and its resulting outputs to our muscles. In order to listen to the still, small voice of the unconscious mind, we need to still the loud monkeys of the conscious mind. In general, I fear, this does not work; many psychiatric efforts to get at the unconscious mind this way have failed to deliver the goods. Nonetheless it remains an interesting ploy. In the paragraphs below, I discuss five ways of stilling the mind: dreams, mental relaxation, meditation, hypnosis, and sensory deprivation.

I consider dreams more fully elsewhere (Chapter 10). They occur when the subject is asleep and are presumably created by a mind free of monkey chatter. They generally appear pretty senseless, and seldom have any clear message: often they seem entirely random. I assume that the unconscious mind invents them, but in the process of pushing them 'upstairs' it censors and disguises them strongly (that deception is presumably part of its strategy for pushing anything upstairs). Psychiatrists have often studied dreams as a way into the unconscious mind, but have needed subtle 'interpretations' to get anywhere.

A very simple way of stilling the monkeys is just by mental relaxation. Many subjects try to relax naturally before, for example, a card-guessing experiment. More dedicated experiments have explored physical relaxation as well. Thus, an electrical myograph (a device for looking for tension in muscles) has been used to encourage the subject to relax totally, and just 'let go' of the body. Ideally, the mind should go blank as well. The outcome seems to be that extrasensory ability is enhanced, detectably but not dramatically.

Another way of quietening those chattering monkeys is meditation. We can probably take it as a more intense and directed form of mental relaxation. Gautama Buddha is said to have meditated for years before suddenly receiving, under a now famous tree, the enlightenment which resulted in the establishment of a major religion. The ancient Indian gurus, sages and yogis explored several techniques of meditation. The earliest written record may be that of Patanjali, who is often considered the founder of the Raja system of yoga. He divided his technique into five initial stages, which appear to have been concerned with eliminating external distraction. The later three stages required increasing concentration on one target image or object. In the final stage, *samadhi*, the attention of the meditator had to be 'totally absorbed' by the target. When that target was finally given up, the mind was completely still.

Modern meditators have sought to monitor their success at stilling the mind by exploiting current electronic brain devices. Thus, electroencephalography puts a number of electrodes around the head, and picks out various electrical rhythms in the brain. One of them, the alpha rhythm, seems linked to sensory input. It is usually broken up by sensory input (e.g. from the eyes) but is maintained by effective meditators. Several investigators in paranormal laboratories have explored meditation to see if it enhances paranormal ability. The results were often encouraging, but were not so striking as to indicate a new and powerful way forward.

Another way of quietening those monkeys is by hypnosis. This was explored in the late 1700s by Friedrich Mesmer, whose theory of 'animal magnetism' was soon superseded. However, in medical hands hypnosis became a way in which a patient could be usefully anaesthetized, but still remain conscious and tractable. In this passive state, the patient essentially abandoned all physiological control to the hypnotist. That patient could be subjected to treatments (such as tooth extraction) that would be painful or troublesome in normal consciousness. Hypnotized subjects have been studied in psychic research to see if the hypnotic state releases useful paranormal abilities. Again, the answer seems to be no, or not much.

Yet another way of 'stilling the mind' may be sensory deprivation. The basic idea is to inhibit as many sensory inputs as you can, so the brain gets as little physical data as possible. It then, perhaps, has to attend to the weak awarenesses that come to it from the unconscious mind. If so, psychic awareness and ability could well rise usefully. The great physicist Richard Feynman is among those who have tried it. He liked the idea of getting 'hallucinations' in the sensory-deprivation tanks employed by John Lilly. Lilly's tanks contained a solution of magnesium sulfate (Epsom Salts: the solution is harmless, but denser than water), held in darkness and silence and close to body heat. When a subject got into such a tank, he or she floated easily, could breathe easily, but received essentially no signals from the eyes or ears, and no thermal information from the skin. The operators could also make the subject a bit dopey with a low dose of the anaesthetic ketamine. Feynman found that he could move his 'ego' about. Most people normally have the sense that 'they' are in their brain, a bit behind the eyes; Feynman could shift his ego around his body, and even outside the room! Feynman had talked to someone who had been in India and had been informed by a guru, and he later called this an 'out-of-body' or OBE experience (I briefly note them in Chapter 10). Feynman managed to have several hallucinations in one of Lilly's sensory-deprivation tanks, but reckoned they came from things he had been thinking about before he went into it. He never reported having any hallucination that seemed to come from outside his own experience.

Many other people have explored sensory deprivation, both for its own sake and as a way of encouraging paranormal experiences. Thus, in the 'ganzfeld' technique (which I discuss in Chapter 8), each eye of the subject is covered by half a ping-pong ball. The result is an unpatterned visual sensation rather like the 'whiteout' dreaded by arctic explorers, in which weather conditions and falling snow totally defeat the visual sense. The subject of the ganzfeld method also has his or her ears saturated by headphones carrying unpatterned 'white noise'. Restricted in this way, the subject seems to be receptive to extrasensory perceptions at greater than chance levels, but not dramatically so.

The unconscious mind as a deceiver

All these techniques ignore something that I feel is central to the unconscious mind. It is inherently a deceiver. It holds on very strongly to anything in its grasp, and whatever it does let up is usually censored or disguised in some way. Hence, of course, the psychiatric art of 'interpreting' dreams—they are never straightforward accounts of whatever is troubling the dreamer. I talk about a typical dream deception in *The Aha! Moment*.[22] Elias Howe, one of the inventors of the sewing machine, had a dream in which he was being led out to execution by warriors with spears—spears which had a hole in the blade, near the point. He woke up, realizing the implication for his sewing machine: the eye of the needle should be near its point! Howe's insight, which must have come from his unconscious mind, determined the whole design of his machine. Indeed, every modern sewing machine follows Howe: it also has a needle with its eye near the point. Freud reckoned that the unconscious mind was tricky and jokey; I go further, and like the biologist Trivers's feel that it is actively misleading. Trivers has claimed that the unconscious mind developed in higher animals to store those dangerous truths that are best kept from other animals. Such worrying truths might include, for example, their position in the pecking order, their hopes of becoming pack leader, and their special friends, enemies, teachers or pupils in the pack. Once these dangerous truths are firmly repressed into the unconscious mind, the animal can lie about them to the other animals. The best liars consciously believe their own lies, and feel quite truthful—this notion is behind George Orwell's terrible technique of 'doublethink', as expounded in his novel *1984*. The unconscious mind exists to hold 'personal political' information safely. This allows the conscious mind, which knows nothing about such worrying realities, to lie about them convincingly. Accordingly, the unconscious mind is not merely weak and easily shouted down: its strategy of deception demands that it be completely silent. That is why, even by the most drastic 'stilling' of the conscious mind, we are almost never aware of it. In human beings, however, I suspect that it may have a further job: it acts as an 'overflow' memory for information that comes in, but cannot easily be held in the limited memory regions of the human brain. However, it probably developed as a form of deception.

Deception seems to be a fundamental part of any information system. In MIT in the 1970s, the first computer was built to be shared by several human users. Its operators were surprised to find that each file needed some sort of personal identifier such as a password, by which each user could protect his or her work from interference from others—possibly from pure jokey malice, but possibly also as a way of gaining some sort of advantage. Those jokers were the forerunners of a whole tribe of malicious 'hackers' whose skill is to penetrate information schemes for gain. We are now seeing the same sort of process at work on the internet, with the development of various 'worms', 'viruses', 'back doors', 'honeypots' and so on. I suspect that in the course of evolution, a large set of ways for extracting modes of information has evolved, together with another whole variety of defensive strategies against it. It interests me, for example, that in the process of digestion (above), all the information in the swallowed food is destroyed before the swallower makes any attempt to use it for personal gain. When I encounter some informational oddity, such as the way that a mentally ill person seems to prefer being ill to becoming aware of the hidden information which might help a psychiatrist (Chapter 8), I ponder that I might have stumbled onto a guard mechanism that makes evolutionary sense. And, of course, my schemes for recovering information from the unknown world via the unconscious mind, have to include strategies against the many deceits and misdirections they are likely to encounter (Chapter 16).

Quite apart from its possible use in guarding against misinformation, the human brain seems not even to be fully used as a holder of true and useful information—as shown by its apparent ability to provide seemingly vacant secondary sites for information lost by a partial brain failure elsewhere (such as a stroke; Chapter 3). Indeed, I have failed to define any believable guess at its storage capacity (Appendix D). I even speculate that we may hold excess information in non-material form, in the unknown world 'outside the diving bell'. This may seem outrageous to readers who automatically assume (as I once did) that everything we know is held in the brain in material form, somewhere in that storage capacity. Yet I like the idea that our unconscious connection to that world may at least allow us to have some access to non-material information. Indeed, I suspect that even some part of our unconscious mind may be there—which is perhaps why it is so hard for psychiatrists to get at. It interests me that the Victorian poet Cosmo Monkhouse, in his poem 'Any Soul to Any Body', takes the physical body as inherently truthful, while the non-material soul often lies. The body sometimes betrays those lies by (for example) blushing or stammering. This fits the notion that it is the non-material element of a person or an animal which is the inherent deceiver.

Accordingly, all dealings with the unconscious mind must expect deceit, and need some way of penetrating it. There are many cases of insights that have turned out entirely fictitious. Kipling's poem 'En-dor' (I refer to it in Chapter 15) has the line: 'Lying spirits perplex us sore'—and his bitter words may have come from life. The most dramatic psychic guessing systems are still mainly wrong. The most successful attempt to get useful information from the non-material world was probably the automatic writing system deployed by Bond and Alleyne (Chapter 15). These investigators found useful information about the Glastonbury Edgar Chapel but never got anywhere with the Loretto Chapel. Even the clever cross-correspondence scheme apparently hatched after death by Myers, Gurney and Sidgwick (Chapter 15) was never unambiguously interpreted. So I feel that while chattering monkeys may be deafening, they are not really fundamental. The voice of the unconscious mind is not so much weak as deceptive. The problem is not just one of removing a strong noise which swamps a weak signal. You need some way of unwrapping or deciphering something which is inherently disguised.

So what should we think about monkey chatter? Several ways of removing it, or at least of reducing it, seem not to have released any significant amount of new psychic ability. My own feeling is that the conscious mind is entirely used to constant monkey chatter, and has its own way of cutting through it to attend to an important new signal. Thus, a sleeping mother may be quite undisturbed by the racket of a passing train, and yet may wake instantly if her baby starts to whimper. Again, I recall waking at once on hearing the odd quiet noise of a falling waterdrop (the roof had started to leak). I have read that one way to be creative is to be the driver on a car journey. The conscious mind is then occupied with many trivial tasks. This keeps it active and out of the way, leaving the unconscious mind to think its own thoughts. The scheme just gives those chattering monkeys something unimportant to chatter about, and lets them get on with it. I feel they are not the main barrier to reaching the unconscious mind. That problem lies deeper. We have to look more carefully at the deceitfulness of the human unconscious, and devise ways of outwitting it, or of correcting its distortions.

Further practical findings which relate to human consciousness

An interesting early experiment was due to William Grey Walter. He had a patient whose brain was exposed (in those days, brain surgery was often conducted under local anaesthesia only; the brain itself has no feeling). Walter was showing the patient a slide show, a series of pictures which could be advanced from one to the next by a carousel mechanism. He told the patient that when he was tired of looking at one picture, he could move to the next by pressing a button. Unknown to the patient, the button did nothing, and the carousel mechanism was connected to part of his brain. He reported to Walter that 'as soon as I decide to look at another picture, the machine advances to it. I never have to press the button!' Clearly, the decision in the patient's brain drove the machine.

Practical brain surgeons often learned a lot about how brains are organized. Thus, some areas seemed to be a store or gatekeeper for memory. If touched, they might elicit a specific memory from the patient; touched again, they might elicit a different one. That specific area seemed to be packed with so densely with memories that the surgeon's touch was not precise enough to trigger any one of them repeatedly. Other areas of the brain were 'silent' and elicited nothing from the patient. They might have been concerned with other brain activities, or perhaps with internal administrative matters (such as the calcium/magnesium ratio of the blood) that never reach conscious attention.

The experimental neurologist Benjamin Libet[26] took Grey Walter's early experiment further. He explored the cerebral response to voluntary wrist movements, and reckoned that detectable intentions arise in the brain before we are conscious of them. His findings seem to imply that we are all robotic zombies driven by pure mechanism. Our consciousness is a mere passive observer ('a kibitzer', as I like to call it) that tags along behind, sees whatever the body does, and maintains the back-dated illusion that it is in control. In reality,our awareness is always a bit behind what we are up to, and is deluding itself. Libet has even measured the length of delay, and makes it a trifle under half a second. He suggests that it gives the brain time to organize a coherent sensory experience out of the frequently distorted input from the senses. Most of the time, of course, we want a true picture of the world around us. But if that picture is too unpleasing, the brain has time to construct a hallucination (I discuss hallucinations in Chapter 10). We habitually back-date our sensory awareness to eliminate that half-second delay.

Libet reckoned that his findings supported the freedom of the will. That half-second between an intention and a conscious awareness of action gives the mind a chance to 'veto' the action. Hence, argued Libet, we do not merely have an illusory sense of free will: we really have it.

5

Methods in Physical Science: Feelings Don't Matter

We have built up a vast amount of scientific knowledge. In the previous chapters, I have briefly sketched out a tiny amount of it, just to provide a framework for my argument about the physical world inside our diving bell. Scientific knowledge is based on careful observations of that world, always followed by publishing them for anyone else to repeat, criticize and argue about. The French poet Valéry wrote in 1932 that 'science is the aggregate of the recipes which always work'. The result is 'public knowledge', testable at any time by anybody who cares to take the trouble. The questioner merely has to repeat the observation or the experiment, and observe the result. It is, or should be, quite independent of the state of mind of that questioner. He or she may be massively ecstatic or massively depressed; it doesn't matter. Either way, the observation will come out the same.

Why Are We Conscious? A Scientist's Take on Consciousness and Extrasensory Perception
David E. H. Jones

ISBN 978-981-4774-32-1 (Hardcover), 978-1-315-16688-9 (eBook)
www.panstanford.com

Einstein reckoned that science depends on two intellectual inventions. One was the axiomatic method of reasoning, invented by the ancient Greeks, and the other was the experimental method, invented during the Renaissance by Galileo. I have claimed that the results then have to be published, for others to repeat, so the 'scientific journal' dedicated to such publications was also an important invention. The outcome is then the 'public knowledge' that makes up science. The experimental method that Galileo expounded is now basic to all science; yet it is a very recent invention. It amazes me, for example, that the laws of falling bodies took so long to become apparent. For millions of years, human beings have been throwing things, both in sport and in warfare. And yet, until Galileo did his famous experiment of dropping a heavy object and a lighter one from the leaning tower of Pisa, nobody had enunciated that most basic gravitational law: the rate of fall of a body does not depend on its weight. That basic truth must have been apparent to anyone who (for example) has even seen a water-splash—big drops and small ones all fall at the same rate. And yet even Aristotle had written that a heavy object falls faster than a light one. The cannon ball, whose flight was of vast military importance, gave a great deal of trouble. Many military men reckoned that it went horizontally for a time, and then fell vertically. It seems obvious to us that it travels in a curve, just like a thrown cricket ball. The curve is flatter than that shown by a cricket ball, because the cannon ball is faster.

The experimental method is a mighty extension of the observations which have been made by philosophers throughout history. Experiment is a powerful way not just of waiting for Mother Nature to produce an effect you can observe, but of setting up some hoop for her to jump through. Of course, Mother Nature is always much cleverer than any experimentalist. Furthermore, she never cheats, and yet the art of devising a convincing experiment, and observing the right outcome, is one of the hardest of practical challenges. Very few scientists have ever been good at it; they are rightly extolled in the history of the subject. Scientific theory, that axiomatic method of reasoning extolled by Einstein, can be even more difficult. The theorist can invent any axioms and follow them through any amount of reasoning of any kind. Yet, if the result is to be scientific, it must ultimately predict something observable, and get it right. Again, it simply does not matter if the mind making the theory is elated, depressed, hopeful, or even deranged. It is only the outcome, the prediction, that matters. And that observation determines the fate of the theory. Perhaps the greatest scientific theory of all was that of Newton, who generalized gravity in about 1700. His theory successfully predicted the positions of the planets and played a huge role in making physics, and indeed all physical science, seem the ultimate arbiter of truth. Yet even Newton did not understand the force of gravity (he needed it as an axiom, but said of it, 'I make no hypothesis,' and indeed, gravity still lies outside many conventions of physics). It was those observations, made by astronomers, which established it as the centrepiece of our scientific account of the public world. They may have been happy, miserable, worried, suspicious or doubtful–none of this mattered. Only the results they found and published matter: and they changed the history of the public world.

Accordingly, the denial that a public world exists at all was a major challenge to philosophy and to science. Such a challenge, which has been since amplified and extended by many other philosophers, was mounted by Locke in 1690. He wrote that all we can know is the contents of our own mind, our sensations and ideas. He claimed that although the physical or sensory world is often alleged to be the source of such sensations and ideas, we can know nothing about it. It is merely a needless duplication of our mental data. Locke was perhaps extending an argument used in the 1000s by the theologian Thomas Aquinas. In the Christian ceremony of communion, the bread and wine consumed by worshippers were held to be transformed into the body and blood of Christ. No change was ever observed in those materials during the ceremony. Aquinas claimed that the appearance of the foodstuffs merely revealed their current 'material accidents', and meant nothing. The bread and wine were in truth miraculously transformed during the ceremony.

Now science is based on the most careful study of physical phenomena. It takes those 'accidents' very seriously indeed. It embodies the ultimate in naïve realism. In physical science, observations are always 'Valerian', independent of the mood of the observer, and the same for almost everybody. But note that 'almost'. Beyond the scientific canon, there are a few people ('star guessers', as I shall call some of them) whose unusual and special ways of feeling and doing things are possibly significant for the world that may be outside our diving bell. Their skills are often regarded as 'psychic'. I discuss in Chapter 6 the way that physical results may differ from 'paranormal' ones. The results of an observation in physical science is (or should be) independent of the mental mood of the observer, while in 'paranormal' studies, that mood can be very important.

It is, of course, true that every physical observation is uncertain, if only because our senses are all different. Fortunately for science, such differences are usually slight and easily allowed for. In one famous case, however, they gave a lot of trouble.

In 1799 the Astronomer Royal Nevil Maskelyne sacked his assistant David Kinnebrook for reporting observations which differed slightly from those of Maskelyne himself. Kinnebrook was not being dishonest or malicious; he just saw things slightly differently from Maskelyne. Any observer has a 'personal equation' which must be allowed for when comparing his or her results with those of anyone else. Each of us lives in a 'private world' unknowable to anybody else, but nearly all such worlds translate, at any rate for our major senses of sight and hearing, into much the same 'public world'. Most observations do not need to be corrected by a 'personal equation' before they can be made public.

Our senses were later scrutinized scientifically by Gustav Fechner. He wrote in 1860 that the smallest noticeable sensory difference is about 1 to 2 percent. Thus one might expect that sort of difference between different observers. This measurement is now part of sensory psychology as the Weber–Fechner law. In chemistry, it often crops up in consistent differences between analysts. Such differences probably arise from a set of consistent habits built up by each individual analyst, perhaps some personal way of making a filtration or of reading a burette. Hence the value of 'standard samples', which should give the same analysis even if analysed by different workers or at different times. This is a good example of the various tricks which experimentalists have evolved to overcome the problems which may arise where human observations differ worryingly. Another is the universal reliance on scientific instruments. We all have different ideas of the temperature, but the reading on a thermometer can be seen and agreed upon by everybody. We are each sensitive to electricity in our own way, but again, the reading on a voltmeter is objective. We may even differ about what we see, but a photograph can be shared by all observers. It is our good fortune that many essentially sporadic and unpredictable events, like those around cosmic rays, happen often enough for single experimental scientists to be able to study them when they occur. As a result, many of their individual reports may be built up into a useful understanding.

However, where a phenomenon is so rare that observations are few and sporadic, trouble often arises. Thus, ball lightning, which we all feel is a simple meteorological phenomenon and part of atmospheric physics, happens so rarely that there is no good theory of it. Nobody understands it. Occasionally, a casual individual encounters it, and whatever that individual has noticed or found interesting is added to the list of 'probable known facts' about it. Such uncommon happenings are seldom discussed by scientists. They acknowledge them reluctantly as 'anecdotal evidence'. This is a sort of scientific code for 'unreliable or unchecked observations'.

Anecdotal evidence

Thus any respectable scientific observation or argument must be published for study, challenge, or verification by others. A small number of observations which cannot be repeated (such as ones about ball lightning) may be taken seriously by scientists, but the vast majority is just dismissed as 'anecdotal evidence'. Yet science is a very small fraction of human knowledge. By far the greatest amount of the things we observe or remember are 'anecdotal evidence'. The physicist Freeman Dyson has written that scientific method is too 'clumsy' to deal with paranormal effects. I disagree. Scientific method sets a very high standard, which few casual or even dedicated observations can live up to. But in my view human experience, which is nearly all anecdotal evidence, and which includes numerous paranormal findings, is too vast to be dismissed just for failing to meet scientific standards.

Nobody has any understanding of the private world inside each of our own minds. Its essential privacy is part of the big general mystery of consciousness. Even what I mean by a simple sensation (say the colour 'red') could be quite unintelligible—not even a colour at all—if reproduced in anyone else's mind. The 'public world' of science contrasts strongly with that private world. We are very lucky that our private worlds all largely 'translate' into a public world that appears much the same for everybody. This good fortune, the naïve realism I salute above, has presumably evolved for every social species. It allows us to cooperate as a tribe, and permits the rise of science as a set of public claims about the physical world. In particular, it permits the rise of 'invisible colleges' all over the earth, in which individual scientists who meet seldom, or never, can each study the same phenomenon.

In the last few hundred years the experimental methods of science have had a massive impact. Every science student absorbs the idea of those 'recipes which are always successful', as Paul Valéry neatly put it. It should give its answer quite independently of the mood of the observer. A good example of a sound Valérian scientific experiment, nowadays part of every syllabus of physics, is the swing of a simple pendulum. This was first studied by Galileo in 1583, after he noticed a suspended lamp swinging in a cathedral and timed it with his pulse. There are at least two interesting things about a pendulum. First, it does not change its time of swing as that swing decreases towards stillness. Second, the time of swing does not depend on the weight of the bob. It does however depend on the force of gravity. That force varies slightly from place to place, and the way it varies over the whole earth has been mapped by pendulum-based gravimeters. The time of a pendulum-swing does, however, depend markedly on the length of the pendulum. Accordingly, a pendulum swings more slowly when it is hot, because heating expands it (hence the value of Harrison's 'grid-iron pendulum', whose length does not rise with temperature). The precise timing of a swinging pendulum has, of course, been the basis of millions of pendulum clocks. Its principles are still echoed in watches and marine chronometers. They also exploit an object undergoing a regular physical change, though one which (unlike a pendulum) does not need a stable gravitational field in a stable direction. Our modern 'quartz crystal' clocks depend on an object which regularly changes shape rather than position, and much faster.

The basic laws of the pendulum are among the 'recipes which are always successful'. They are simply what they are, and just wait to be discovered. They are the same for all experimenters, and fully part of the physical world. They depend solely on the equipment as set up. They do not depend at all on the mood, attitude, expectations or mental capacity of the experimenter. That pugnacious biochemist J. B. S. Haldane once claimed to be a 'practising atheist'. He explained that his assumption during any scientific experiment was that no miracle or divine intervention would interfere with the result or his observation of it. In that sense, every physical scientist is a 'practising atheist', whose assumption is that his mental attitude to his experiment and observation is also irrelevant to its result.

One of my treasures is a 'Stanton' chemical balance of the type I used as a chemical undergraduate. I suppose that when it was designed, it was at the cutting edge of chemical research. By the 1960s it was so out of date that it was downgraded to undergraduate use. In modern terms it is a museum piece. And yet it records the weight of a sample in a very Valérian way. It is utterly objective. Like any reliable scientific instrument, it is quite unaffected by the mental approach of the user. If it gives the weight of a sample as (say) 17.5142 grams, my strongest hope will not raise the figure to 17.5143 grams. My most desperate despair will not lower it to 17.5141 grams. Another observer would always agree with me. Paul Valéry, with Henry Stanley and Albert Harrington (who in 1946 founded the firm that made it), would be proud of that balance. And yet this book is largely about observations which are not all Valérian. Thus the great Victorian scientist William Crookes devised a special balance which could be deflected by thoughts from Daniel Dunglas Home, a medium of the day. Fortunately for science, such effects—even if they are not a clever fraud—are extremely rare!

All science has been built up by chance-bound observers like myself, and instruments like that honest Stanton balance have been developed for them to handle. We all need, and take for granted, the objectivity of experimental physical results. It may well take a genius to invent an experiment, and literary skill to publish its description. But thereafter any reader, whether a collaborator or a rival or an independent worker, should be able to repeat it and verify it. In the early days of science, this was generally true. Pioneers such as Dalton and Lavoisier worked like this. They did new experiments by themselves, described them and wrote about them, and constructed theories on what they had found. Their disciples repeated and extended such experiments, and broadened the theories.

These days, many things are very different. A great originator may have a brilliant new idea, but often many co-workers and many years are required to explore and extend it. Thus the mighty American physicist Ernest Lawrence invented that clever accelerator for nuclear particles, the cyclotron. His original machine of 1931 fitted on a laboratory bench: its magnet was about 28 centimetres across. Anybody could make one like it, and check that Lawrence's idea made sense, and that his findings were sound and repeatable. Its latest exemplification is in Geneva, the CERN Large Hadron Collider, which occupies a tunnel about 9 km in diameter. Many of its staff are not scientists at all, but technicians with the job of (for example) tracking down leaks, or checking that amplifiers are working to specification. In psychology, a very different branch of science, and pioneers such as Sigmund Freud and Carl Jung (I mention them in Chapter 8), studied single human subjects. A modern psychological research often considers a huge cohort of subjects, who are frequently told some lie about what the experiment is about. The researchers examine the responses of their subjects by subtle statistical methods to deduce some aspect of human nature and its variation in their subjects.

Modern research is seldom individual. Most scientific papers these days have at least two authors. Some research activities require big teams (for example, the Large Hadron Collider and much of collective psychology). I am saddened by this, and have a sort of nostalgia for the old days of individual thought and enterprise. Valéry's ideal single experiment is rare in current cutting-edge research.

One result of present-day scientific collective enterprise, and the expense and organization needed to advance it even slightly, is that its conclusions are often presented to the non-scientist as a sort of unchallengeable intellectual diktat. Thus, few of us could check for ourselves the existence of the Higgs boson, or the recession of the galaxies. We rely on the findings of those teams of specialists. We accept their dominance, just as we accept that of the great figures of the arts.

Sadly, while science itself is repeatably Valérian, the technology based on it is often so complicated that it is always liable to fail. Typically, some component breaks down. A lecturer I heard once explored this notion. He asked, 'How much would you pay for petrol if it came with a guarantee that your car would never go wrong?', and guessed that we might pay twice the usual price. Again, I once read of a missionary who asked a tribesman why his tribe went in for drums, telepathy, and so on, as a means of communicating. 'Because we don't have the telephone' came the reply. This unexpected response has, I feel, a message for all of us. In physical science, we expect that any published experiment will always work.

Incidentally, the objectivity and the predictability, so important in scientific recipes, are also crucial features of civilized life. One of the greatest of human inventions was the idea of a written law. In some ways it parallels the 'laws of nature' established by physical science. Our earliest example of such a law may have been inscribed on a Persian stone in about 1800 BC by scribes working for the Babylonian king Hammurabi. Before that, the law (if it existed at all) was very flexible. It does not even exist in animal tribes, which are often dominated and controlled by whatever enters the minds of the gang of thugs at the top. An anthropologist studying the primitive human tribes in South America once asked a member of such a tribe what he most admired about civilized life. The respondent ignored all the technical gadgetry of civilization: he replied, 'The Law.' The impartiality of a set of universal rules seemed to him far superior to the biased and often unpredictable decisions of tribal leaders. When in the 1960s I was researching for a chemical Ph.D., the laboratory also contained a Pakistani chemist. He was greatly impressed by a British news item in which the daughter of Winston Churchill was arrested on a traffic charge. The judge said, 'You may be the daughter of the greatest living statesman but you cannot escape the Law!' My Pakistani friend implicitly contrasted this state of affairs with the situation in Pakistan, in which those connected with the government often managed to slip out of the obligations which enmeshed ordinary citizens. Of course, even today lots of societies set up forms of escape for people near the top. By contrast, many democracies seem to have evolved a sort of unwritten 'civic religion' which imposes expectations not only on the citizens, but on the authorities: it limits what they can do. One of its major terms is a strong restraint on financial corruption. Transparency International even maintains and publishes a 'corruption perception index', in which nations are judged on their degree of corruption. It defines corruption as the misuse of public power for private benefit. In 2013 it ranked the United States of America 19th and the U.K. 14th out of 176 countries on its list. I have read of many so-called kleptocracies in which the government almost openly spends public money to benefit its leaders. The ideal of a written law which applies equally to everyone is still largely unrealised.

Scientific education

Normal scientific education invites its students to learn only to pay attention to their experiment or the reading on their apparatus. For most of us, this makes excellent sense. I have remarked earlier in this chapter how I have been quite unable to alter the reading on a chemical balance by any mental effort, and (like most of us) I have never come across any object which did not seem completely obedient to whatever physical forces were acting upon it. Good science students soon learn by painful practice the art of doing an experiment. They come to understand that an experiment is not just a meaningless exercise in manipulating bits of gear, but is a question put to Mother Nature. They then have to learn the way of writing about it so that someone else with the same sort of background can repeat it and get the same result. It can take many years to develop the skills that every researcher needs.

This laboratory experience matters. Even the most abstruse scientific theoreticians will have picked it up. We have all learned to beware of the man who has no practical experience of a subject, but 'knows all about it' from reading. I fear that the only useful current way to pick up experimental skill is the often-derided method 'sit by Nellie'. It is clumsy and slow, but it works. The learner picks up, not only the 'written rules' of the job, but many important 'unwritten rules' needed for skill, ability and even flair. Most of us have learned our job in this way; it is universal in apprenticeship and in the tricky art of learning how to do scientific research. I am still waiting, without much hope, for a way of transmitting ability from one mind to another without writing, reading, listening to speech, screen-watching, or sitting by Nellie.

Some powerful scientists, however, may understand experimental skills, but never get to be good at them. They perhaps become theoreticians, adept with the notebook and at home with the argument, but a mighty nuisance in the laboratory. One famous Nobel Prize–winning physical theoretician has even made a jocular claim about his disruptive physical style. He has stated that he could wreck any experiment merely by entering the laboratory. A commanding experimenter has even attributed the sudden implosion of his vacuum equipment to the way the theoretician's train momentarily stopped at a local station.

6

Methods in Paranormal Science: Feelings Do Matter

The above discussion may seem to imply that physical science laboratories should all be much alike. In practice, they vary greatly. Some, such as the Bell Telephone Laboratories in the United States, and the Cavendish Laboratory in Cambridge in the United Kingdom, acquired great reputations for the novelty and originality of their achievements. This may largely have been self-generated. Once an establishment has acquired a high reputation, it often tends to make it higher still. As in any sort of institution, high-class laboratories attract high-class scientists, and gain still more as a result. And yet an experiment in physical science does not depend on the experimenter. Possibly because of some personal theory he is exploring, such an experimenter may set up and try out a highly unusual original experiment and observe its outcome with care. A good example is the cavity magnetron, invented at the U.K. Birmingham University

Why Are We Conscious? A Scientist's Take on Consciousness and Extrasensory Perception
David E. H. Jones

ISBN 978-981-4774-32-1 (Hardcover), 978-1-315-16688-9 (eBook)
www.panstanford.com

in 1942 by the physicists John Randall and Harry Boot. This highly original device could generate watts of power at gigahertz frequencies. It was invented during the Second World War, and transformed radar: it became the RAF's most cherished secret. It did not depend in the least on the mental state of Randall and Boot. Indeed, had the design been published, it would have been very easy to copy. Any experiment in physical science, however ingenious and unusual, is published in due course; the whole idea is that it can then be copied and verified by another worker. That worker may have an entirely different state of mind to the inventor, and perhaps could never have invented the design himself or herself. My feeling is that some prompting from the unconscious mind of the inventor stimulates the new conscious idea. In Chapters 16 to 18 of this book, I imagine experiments in which the unknown world outside our diving bell can be explored without employing a human mind as part of the equipment.

However, at present a 'paranormal' laboratory is quite unlike a physical one. The outcome of a paranormal experiment often depends crucially on the attitude of its workers. Frequently its findings cannot be repeated in another laboratory. They seem to turn on the personalities of the people carrying them out, or those of the experimental 'subjects'. In stark contrast to the repeatable, Valérian nature of experiments in physical science, many of the 'paranormal' experiments that I want to discuss seem very dependent upon the mood of the experimenter. A card guesser, for example, guesses less successfully if he or she is bored or depressed, and as the session progresses, his or her skill often declines steadily, although it may perk up towards the end. Much depends on the subtle, uncontrollable 'atmosphere' of the work.

Any thinker musing on a paranormal experiment has to accept this mental dependence. Physical science often gains from a passive attitude–let Mother Nature get on with it! Even so, a good physical scientist always does a new experiment several times, at least to look for possible variations. Thus a biologist always has to bear in mind that animals vary greatly in their individuality, so the one he is investigating may be unusual in some way or another. 'Control' experiments, in which the crucial variables are carefully kept the same, are important in all science. Even psychological, and especially paranormal, experiments usually employ them. Even so, the personalities of the subjects and the experimenters (and their unconscious minds, which we can never know about) may have a great influence on the outcome.

In the late 1920s and throughout the 1930s, Joseph Rhine at the Paranormal Laboratory in Duke University, North Carolina, USA, felt that his whole operation greatly gained from its mood. He extolled its infectious and enthusiastic atmosphere. I suspect that Rhine also gained from the happy accident that several 'star guessers' came to work there. His book of 1934, *Extra-Sensory Perception* (ESP), spurred a lot of interest. However, later attempts to replicate his findings, maybe in a less enthusiastic atmosphere, and with fewer 'star' guessers, did not always succeed. (Duke University later severed its connections with the Paranormal Laboratory, but it continues its work as an independent institution, the Rhine Research Center.) In the 1950s and 1960s Gertrude Schmeidler looked into the correlation of the mental attitude of paranormal subjects with their results. She divided her subjects into 'sheep' who believed in the possibility of extrasensory perception, and 'goats' who denied it. She found that in general 'sheep' show higher paranormal scores than 'goats'. 'Goats' might even score negatively, below chance, as if sensing a truth but avoiding it. So much depends on mental attitude! Thus Eileen Garrett, one of the greatest mediums of the 1900s, visited Rhine's Laboratory in 1934, and took a card-guessing test. To everybody's surprise, including her own, she scored at ordinary 'chance' levels. Only when she had escaped the boredom of the test, and had given it some sort of human emotional interest, did her special powers emerge. Her 'paranormal powers' depended on her feelings, and behaved quite differently from the scientific 'recipes which always work'.

This sort of mental effect can often be very inhibitory. I have read of psychic researchers who fear that they personally can inhibit paranormal experiments entirely—despite being consciously all in favour of the work. Such a researcher may design an experiment, but will then depart and leave it to be actually carried out by more enthusiastic and less inhibited underlings. This agrees with the notion that positive paranormal results (unlike physical ones) may depend on the mental attitude of the researcher. In this case, perhaps the skepticism or disbelief of the researcher is hidden in his or her unconscious mind. The person cannot hope to get at it, challenge it, or even know about it. It might need a psychiatric investigation to bring it up to consciousness (and such investigations do not always work).

I have not read of any study of this effect. Does the inhibitor have to leave the district, or merely the building? Does the effect decline with the distance, or with the square of the distance, or by any other law, or by any form of screening? My sense is that distance or physical screening must have some effect: otherwise just one skeptic anywhere could inhibit every paranormal experiment everywhere.

The importance of mental attitude in 'paranormal' work is strongly exemplified by an account from the 1970s of an experiment discussed by I. M. Owen and M. H. Sparrow (Conjuring up Philip[30]) conducted by the Toronto Society for Psychical Research. Workers in that Society planned to invent an entirely fictitious 'ghost', which they called 'Philip'. They invented a completely imaginary history for Philip and hoped ultimately to obtain a visible apparition of him. (They failed, in the sense that they never got anything visible, but they were able to interrogate Philip, and obtain rappings and dramatic movements of the table they sat around.)

The Toronto group originally had 14 members, but some withdrew, leaving 8 'regulars'. None of the eight claimed any psychic ability—indeed, one idea behind the formation of the group was that a group of normal people might have the power of one 'psychic'. (Many people have been dismayed by the erratic and unpredictable nature of any sort of individual psychic power. They have mused that the effect is humanly statistical, so that a large number of ordinary people thinking together could produce repeatable and convincing results. I have even proposed the idea myself[19], but a few large-scale studies have not been promising.) The Toronto workers took a long time to create their fictitious ghost: in fact it took a year of joint meditation to bring 'Philip' to life. Towards the end of that year, they were greatly influenced by a doctrine expounded by Colin Brookes-Smith[6] in the *Journal of the Society for Psychical Research*. He extolled Kenneth Batcheldor's theories of the sort of mental attitude that encouraged the emergence of physical phenomena in a group situation. Batcheldor felt that the group must be able to accept the fact that that paranormal phenomena are happening without expressing, inwardly or outwardly, astonishment or disbelief. A skeptical attitude could effectively stop the phenomena. A typical Victorian séance had a relaxed and even childish atmosphere, which helped to dispel such skepticism, and more or less by accident, the Toronto group came to adopt it. One member of that group even extolled its childish rejection of skepticism: 'If I want it to happen, it will!'

In group work, said Batcheldor, it seems important that there should be no special 'leader' or medium responsible, and thus there needs to be an alternative focus for group attention. For the Toronto group, this was the table around which they were sitting. The group in effect personalized the table, addressed it as Philip, and were able to get it to rap and move. In a strange way, it was like a separate person. This accepting atmosphere of 'heightened expectancy' made them open-minded and prepared to believe that paranormal results could be produced. That year of joint meditation had given them total rapport with each other, the ability to relax in each other's company, even a feeling that they formed a close family. The Toronto group discovered that this 'solidarity' had to be kept up. If the group became at all hesitant, the raps and movements of the table became weaker. But by building up a consistent and shared notion of Philip's story and character, they eliminated the individual deviations that could inhibit their findings. Philip gave them no information they had not devised beforehand—they seem not to have tried to elicit any.

They called their results 'psychokinesis by committee'. The invented ghost Philip was in effect responsible for everything, and no member of the group had to bother about events. Nobody in the group had to concentrate on anything. Even visitors commented on how natural it all looked. My impression is that the group had learned how to create the right frame of mind in which psychokinetic effect could occur.

There are several stories of information existing in the unknown world outside our diving bell, and later being retrieved from it. Indeed, it is an important theme in this book that lots of information exists in that unknown world, and we may be able to acquire some of it (I suggest possible ways of doing this in Chapter 16). Elizabeth

Mayer's book *Extraordinary Knowing*[27] gives several examples of people knowing things that in principle they should not know. She seems not to expound any theory of where that knowledge might come from. My speculation is that all such knowledge comes from the unknown world via some unconscious mind. It might come in from another human mind (telepathy, Chapter 8), or directly from the unknown world by clairvoyance or precognition. My favourite example of information retrieved from the unknown world is that of Bond and Alleyne. They obtained information about the Edgar Chapel at Glastonbury apparently from the memory of dead monks (Chapter 15). This suggests that human information may survive bodily death. I have noted the almost universal belief in some sort of survival after death (e.g. Chapter 12), and I like the idea that some human information could survive the death of the body. This notion is encouraged by the story of Myers, Gurney and Sidgwick (Chapter 15). It is even further extended by psychiatric claims of apparent memories of 'previous lives', 'past persons' and even of the 'race memory' and 'animal memory' sometimes reported by patients. Thus I have been greatly moved by an account reported by a patient of the fearful feelings of an ancestor while he was being executed. I cannot imagine any biological way in which his final moments could be recorded and passed on to a distant descendant. And yet I am unwilling to dismiss the story as pure fantasy. In Chapters 8 to 11 I sketch numerous paranormal effects which seem to have been experimentally observed. They are largely condensed from a handbook of parapsychology[37].

7

The Physical Properties of the Unknown World Outside Our Diving Bell

In Chapter 1, I assume that the unknown world outside our diving bell occupies the same space as the physical one, and is superposed on it. We are in a sense immersed in it, just as we are immersed in physical space; I take the two worlds as very weakly coupled. In this chapter, I consider what limitations may be placed on the unknown world by that superimposition. My suggestions are, of course, scientific guesswork, but they may at least provide a framework for thinking about that world.

What is it made up of?

I simply cannot guess an answer to this question. I guess that it has, like the world we know about, information in some form, energy in some form and matter in some form.

Why Are We Conscious? A Scientist's Take on Consciousness and Extrasensory Perception
David E. H. Jones

ISBN 978-981-4774-32-1 (Hardcover), 978-1-315-16688-9 (eBook)
www.panstanford.com

An item of information, such as a divination of the future, a sudden insight, a correct guess, a piece of knowledge that may originally have come from someone now dead, occasionally enters a human mind. It is worth wondering whether it comes from that unknown world. Some of it may be associated with objects in that world, which 'know' something. It also may exist in some detached, non-material form, such as ordered radiation. Whatever form that information may take, it is often in some way accessible to a human unconscious mind. I assume the unknown world has some form of energy, which seems to be implied by the rappings which it originates, and by the strange energetic operations of poltergeists and the alleged levitations caused by mediums. It may contain some form of matter, too—this seems implied by my notion that the unknown world has a temperature. In the physical world we know about, temperature is just the average velocity-energy of the local molecules. I have no idea what it may correspond to in the unknown world. If that world has matter as a continuum rather than a system of particles, it will be quite different. Objects may also exist in that world, made up from these ingredients in some unknown way. In this text I simply call them all 'entities', but avoid making any more detailed structural guesses.

The temperature of the unknown world

What is the temperature of the unknown world? This is a strange sort of question to begin with. However, it happens to be the one which got me thinking; I have mused about it both in *Nature*[18] and in *Chemistry World*[20]. Temperature is the average velocity-energy possessed by a molecule. It is not obvious that a world that is not made of molecules can even have a temperature. Yet I muse that the world outside our diving bell may possess some form of energy.

One of the most fundamental facts of physics is that two objects in even feeble contact will equilibrate to the same temperature. I therefore imagine that over the lifetime of the universe (which I take to be about 13 billion years) the unknown world will have come to share the same average temperature as the physical world on which it is superposed. The two may be very weakly coupled, indeed they may almost be separate, but during those long ages they ought to have reached thermal equilibrium. It may make sense to imagine that the unknown world has some sort of temperature, and it is interesting to guess what it might be.

Unfortunately, the average temperature of the physical world is itself badly known. Let us neglect the possible existence and unknown temperature of 'dark matter'. The average temperature of the physical universe is then probably dominated, not by its relatively few and widely spaced hot stars, but by its vast content of cold interstellar gas. A good guess for that average temperature might be about 10 K. The cosmic microwave background sets a strong lower limit. It is at about 3 K and pervades the whole universe, so no natural object can be colder than that.

The objects which we handle in the kitchen and the laboratory are usually much hotter than 10 K, typically about 290 K. Let us suppose that they are indeed very weakly coupled to the unknown world. Then, any object which was totally thermally isolated and deprived of any physical source of heat, would slowly cool down. It would creep towards the temperature of the unknown world with which it was still weakly in contact. That cooling might be smallest for a material with the least coupling. Conversely, an object with some connection with the unknown world might cool towards its temperature more rapidly. Indeed, the rates of cooling of various types of material might give useful clues to the nature of that unknown world. Joule's theory that heat was a form of energy did not at first convince the scientific world because, as Thomas Graham remarked in 1847 that 'he only had hundredths of a degree to prove his case by'. Later, of course, Joule's theory was well established. It is now a fundamental part of science, and the unit of energy is the joule. This story encourages me, for my speculation here is even feebler. It depends on millionths of a degree of slow cooling of very carefully isolated physical objects, and nobody has even looked for it. But if that slow cooling were ever established, it would be a very fundamental way of showing the existence of the unknown world. My conjecture that different physical objects might cool at different rates is even wilder. But if a sensitive enough cooling technique were ever developed, it might be worth looking for.

J. T. McMullan of the School of Physical Sciences at the New University of Ulster in Northern Ireland, in a letter[28] published in 1971 in the *Journal of the American Society for Psychical Research*, suggested that a poltergeist might get energy from cooling the room. A ghost may indeed cool the room; indeed there are many reports of such coolings, though it is not obvious whether they report a real thermometric effect or a human feeling of coldness. Nonetheless McMullan's notion is contrary to the laws of thermodynamics. These laws apply strongly within the physical world but, of course, may not apply to exchanges of energy between the physical world and the unknown one. McMullan truly points out that a room has energy by virtue of its temperature above absolute zero. The laws of thermodynamics, however, imply that you cannot get at that energy by cooling the room. In fact you cannot cool it at all without supplying energy (this is why a refrigerator needs power to drive it). To get useful energy you need not a temperature, but a temperature difference.

Our current technology overwhelming gets its energy by burning the combustible portions of the planet–coal, oil, and latterly gas. This burning creates a temperature difference we can use. All our usual heat engines have not only a hot 'boiler' but also a colder 'condenser', which in the case of an internal combustion engine is just its radiator and the atmosphere which receives its exhaust. The second law of thermodynamics demands that temperature difference–which is why land-locked power stations have cooling towers. The media keep reminding us about the growing energy crisis, and make many absurd claims about a switch to forms of 'renewable energy', such as solar power, wind power, and so on. Meanwhile, our thermal circumstances are made worse by the fact that all normal technical operations release 'waste heat'. Not one of them is thermally efficient. Bending, cutting, industrial chemistry, illuminating, and so on, all release heat as waste. This is dispersed into the environment, sometimes casually and sometimes by special radiators.

Bond and Alleyne (Chapter 15), who acquired architectural information about the long-destroyed Glastonbury Abbey by automatic writing, encountered problems with temperature. During a very cold spell of weather in January 1908, they failed in their efforts. Whatever entity wrote their automatic script complained 'Frigidus sum' (Latin for 'I am cold'). That complaint may refer to the coldness of the human arms through which data had to be transferred. If it refers to the world from which the writing came, and if that world was the unknown one I am musing about, this contradicts my assumption that that world is very cold. An entity in that world would be unconcerned with the temperature in this one. For the moment I will maintain my thesis, and continue to assume that my posited unknown world is much colder than our physical world of warm or cold weather.

McMullan's thermal notion suggests some interesting technical possibilities. If there were any good way of disposing of heat by dumping it into the cold parts of the world, we could not merely get rid of unwanted waste heat; we could generate any amount of new energy. We would merely have to use our local environment as a boiler, and a cold bit of the world as a condenser. If we could reach outside our physical diving bell to get at it, the unknown world at about 10 K could make a useful condenser. Sadly, I cannot even see any way of getting at it at all, let alone turning it into a condenser. Even so, I like the idea of generating power from the temperature differences provided by nature.

The duration of the unknown world

What is its duration? In this text I take the spatial region potentially accessible to us about 10^{70} km^3 (Chapter 2). Beyond this region, the galaxies are receding faster than the speed of light, so that we can never observe them. Its time scale is even more uncertain. The current 'Big Bang' theory of the start of the physical world is somewhat based on that claimed recession of the galaxies. It assumes that the physical world started as a tiny object about 13 billion years ago. This view clearly does not apply to the unknown world. It might have started later or earlier, or might indeed have extended 'from everlasting to everlasting' as the religious quotation claims. If, as this text assumes, we take it as weakly coupled to the physical world, the time of interest to us is about 13 billion years into the past, and perhaps an equal time into the future.

The dimensionality of the unknown world

What dimensions does it have? To be neatly superposed on the physical world, it needs the same dimensions as that physical world, i.e. three of space plus one of time. However, physical space may have more dimensions, at least spatial ones. Some 'superstring theorists' want it to have ten or even eleven spatial dimensions. They claim that all except three are curled up so tightly we cannot be aware of them. If you imagine a hose-pipe, for example, it may look from a distance like a simple line. But if you look at it closely, you will see that it has an extra dimension, and is really an extended closed circle. That circle is curled up and very small. I have read the claim that physical space is like this too, with all but three dimensions unobservable. My sense is that the whole idea is fanciful. Superstring theorists want their ten or eleven dimensions not for any inherently logical or spatial reason, but just to make their theories work. I have mused (Chapter 17) that extremely long distances in physical space might be neatly bridged in the space outside our diving bell.

I return to the possible spatial connections between the physical and unknown worlds. If that world had fewer spatial dimensions than the physical world, say by being flat or linear, there would be large sections of the physical world in which it did not exist. In such regions nothing would be conscious (if consciousness depends on contact with it: Chapter 1), nobody could pray or have any sense of enlightenment (if such activities also depend on it), no psychic or paranormal effects could be observed, and so on. I know of no such regions. Even so, it is possible to assert that the unknown world is somehow 'closer' to the physical one in certain locations. Thus the ancient Greek oracle at Delphi was a special cavern, in which an oracular person could achieve important insights. A temple was built over it. The body of St Cuthbert of Lindisfarne was one of the holy relics being moved by Northumbrian monks in the 1000s. The oxen hauling his coffin in a wagon stopped at a spot in a curve of the River Wear, and refused to move on. The monks felt that this was a sign of local holiness, and implied that that he should be buried there. Later the site was dignified by the erection of Durham Cathedral, one of the glories of English architecture. The old town of Glastonbury in Southern England has been a special religious site for centuries. It is one of the (many) places in which Jesus of Nazareth may have lived before his ministry. It may still retain its significance; the holy Shambhala site of Hinduism has been identified with it.

If the unknown world had more spatial dimensions than physical space, the two worlds would again match badly. Much of it would be inaccessible to the physical world. My assumption that the two are superposed and have the same average temperature, would be even less convincing. To make the argument work at all, I would have to assume that the whole hypervolume of unknown space was being stirred so effectively for so much of its time that each element of it spent enough time in contact with the physical world to acquire its average temperature.

We usually assume that normal physical space has three dimensions and contains objects made of particles. The unknown world may be quite different, although I have mused about spaces which also contain particulate matter but have other dimensions.[23] The puzzle makes no obvious sense. Physical space seems to have three dimensions of space and one of time, but logic would seem just as satisfied by (say) ninety-seven and thirteen.

However, it seems feasible to guess the unknown world is less bound to space than the physical one. Thus in Chapter 17 I speculate that if we could enter the unknown world and leave it again, we might be able to travel many light-years while avoiding the conventional technology of space travel. Most of the physical phenomena I discuss in Chapters 8 to 11 have strong local elements (the collective unconscious,if it exists, may be an exception; telepathy may be another, and so may guessing cards better than chance). Even so, local effects can sometimes seem very strong. Certain unusual people have been able to fog nearby chemical film but not distant film (Chapters 6 and 9), and some researchers seem to inhibit paranormal investigations so much that they have to leave the experiment.

I am also interested in the 'time' dimension of the space outside our diving bell. Within it, we move steadily and unalterably through time, despite our freedom to move through our three accessible spatial dimensions. The unknown world outside our diving bell may have more temporal freedom. I have read in theological texts that the world as viewed by God is 'outside time' completely, so that He knows both our past and our future. This implies that the past and the future both exist somewhere. The same sort of temporal freedom may apply to the unknown world. This is a strange idea, but seems supported by the decay of scientific determinism and the existence of quantum-mechanically 'uncaused events' (Appendix C). It also gains some support from paranormal experiments which imply that a card guess may be a better fit, not to a card being presented now, but to one about to come in three seconds or so. It is also supported by the 'divinations' of one medium who could apparently predict events years in the future (Chapter 14). Sleep-dreams about the future have even been recorded! So my musings that the unknown world has more temporal freedom than ours, and may have information about the past and the future in it, may make some sort of sense. This notion encourages me to propose that 'star guessers', who guess a bit better than chance, may get their information telepathically from the past or future (Chapter 14).

My sense is that the unknown world must have at least one dimension of time. If it had none, it would be entirely static, and would always be the same. Its entities could never change. A ghost could never move (which would make a nonsense of haunting), and the many recorded instances in which it has caused changes in the physical world would be even more puzzling than they already are.

One inviting notion is that 'time travel' may be possible in the unknown world. This would explain its apparent access to information about the past and the future. I can put forward the idea that the unknown world has two or more temporal dimensions. Maybe travel in one or more of them is possible? I cannot understand this, nor make any useful deductions from it. More or less by default, the discussion in this book takes the unknown world outside our diving bell as simply superposed everywhere on the physical one, both in the three dimensions of space and the one of time. Nonetheless, I remain open to the idea that it may have some sort of spatial and temporal flexibility, and could allow us access to information from the past or from the future. I explore these notions in Chapter 14.

What velocities are there in the unknown world?

I assume that the entities in that world can move around in its space, just as objects do in the physical world. So it makes sense to guess at the sort of velocities with which they do it. The notion in Chapter 10, that most human ghosts do not appear to us because they are in interstellar space, also implies some sort of movement in that world. I like the idea, but it says nothing about the range of velocities possible for such movement.

I am tempted to take the physical world as a useful analogy. It has no absolute velocities but many relative ones. In the laboratory, a typical molecular speed relative to the apparatus might be a few hundred $m \cdot s^{-1}$. Astronomical objects often go rather faster. Thus the Sun itself rotates with our galaxy, and in addition may have an individual motion of its own. Its average velocity relative to nearby matter may be something like 10,000 $m{\cdot}s^{-1}$, say a solar diameter every few minutes. If by analogy the unknown world is similar, the entities in that world might also have an average velocity of about 10,000 $m{\cdot}s^{-1}$—though doubtless with a huge range on either side. Now the physical world consists essentially of a vast volume of cold interstellar gas. An entity in the unknown world, moving at 10,000 $m{\cdot}s^{-1}$ through that cold gas, and making even weak contact with it, would spend almost all its time in that weak contact. Every 10,000 years or so that entity might spend a few minutes passing through, and weakly contacting, a hot star. My guess is that this weak coupling to a very brief source of great heat would have almost no effect. Its average thermal experience of the physical world would essentially be that of cold interstellar gas. If it acquires a temperature (as I surmise in Chapter 7), it should be that of the cold gas, maybe 10 K.

What is the typical size of the entities in the unknown world?

The question is so obvious that I cannot avoid it. In my discussion of velocities in the unknown world, I implicitly assumed an entity much smaller than a star. And yet I am unwilling to make any guesses about size. My sense is that the entities in the unknown world do not have a size. Like a physical gas, they have no specific shape or size, though they may have some sort of position.

What sort of entities might there be in the unknown world?

In the above discussion of that world, its properties and possible contents, I have been dodging this question. As a scientist, I cannot answer it at all, though in Chapter 12

I note that the unknown world has many similarities to the informal world seemingly believed in by many non-scientific people. If that world is outside time, or more flexible about it than our physical clocks and calendars, it might hold information not only from the present physical world, but from its past or its future. It might include powerful predictions, such as scientific findings which have not yet been made, or data from the past which we have irretrievably lost. I like the idea of retrieving some of that information.

What information is contained in the unknown world?

This is an important question. Later in this book (Chapters 15 to 18) I discuss ways of getting information from the unknown world, and imagine instrumental methods which might be developed to do it. Information in the physical world is often associated with objects in it, sometimes as memories stored in a brain or a computer disk. In such cases a specific code is used to associate each item of information with a specific arrangement of physical structure, such as the size, shape or magnetic character of a component. An older way of storing information uses marks on paper, typically as writing or print. But these days, information often occurs without any physical manifestations—as in the frequencies and modulations of electromagnetic waves. I cannot guess the sort of ways in which information might occur in the unknown world. Much may be associated with or under the control of entities within it, but some (such as telepathic messages) may be a pure signal. There does not seem to be any special limit equivalent to the speed of light—which in the physical world limits the rate at which information can be transmitted.

8

Observed Effects of the Unconscious Mind and the Unknown World. 1: Mental Effects

UP TO THIS POINT, MY BOOK has been very remote from reality. I have discussed briefly a little of what science seems to have discovered about the physical world. I have deplored its inability to find anything about the only thing of which we are directly aware–human consciousness. I have extolled the unconscious mind, about which we know so little. I have proposed an unknown world, which occupies the same space as the physical space that we are aware of, but which no scientific instrument has been made to detect, and which indeed has never been detected. However, I now want to go beyond this discouraging remoteness. In the next four chapters I shall outline many items of physical evidence in favour of my claims. I feel that despite their almost universal failure to abide by the

Why Are We Conscious? A Scientist's Take on Consciousness and Extrasensory Perception
David E. H. Jones

ISBN 978-981-4774-32-1 (Hardcover), 978-1-315-16688-9 (eBook)
www.panstanford.com

repeatable, Valérian scientific method, the vast number of human 'anecdotal evidence' observations deserve to be taken seriously!

Many of the effects I describe seem to have demanded some sort of explanation for decades, but have never been provided with one. Others seem relatively dubious. It is hard for me as a scientist even to admit their existence, let alone to take them seriously. Some may even have been set up by fraud and trickery; yet they have all also been supported by competent and detached observers. I feel that any effect that is reported by many people deserves to be noted. Each of my four chapters of physical evidence has at least one very significant topic. I mention many others which seem in my favour, including some I do not understand at all.

Psychiatry

The unconscious mind is central to current psychiatry, which is at least in part a sort of scientific attempt to study it. I call it 'sort of' because, firstly, it is a method of alleviating human illness and is therefore a technology rather than a science, and secondly, psychiatric theory has so little critical scientific backing that it has been strongly denounced by many scientists. Thus the biochemist Peter Medawar wrote: 'Considered in its entirety, psychoanalysis won't do. It is an end product, moreover, like a dinosaur or a zeppelin; no better theory can ever be erected on its ruins, which will remain for ever one of the saddest and strangest of all landmarks in the history of twentieth century thought.'

The great psychiatrist Sigmund Freud divided the human mind into several divisions. This text divides it into four. At the top is Freud's 'super-ego', which holds the personal ideals of the subject. Below that is the ordinary consciousness, Freud's 'ego', which is what we are commonly aware of. It holds the things in our ordinary consciousness, and the awareness of the nearby physical world, as brought in by our senses. It holds our social reactions towards the other human beings with whom we are currently interacting. Below that is the subconscious mind, with which I feel we retain good contact. It holds our vast array of skills and memories, and all the things that we are not thinking about or aware of at the moment, but can bring very rapidly into consciousness if the need develops. Crucially, it holds our linguistic vocabulary, which can easily contain thousands of words and their meanings. We can deploy these almost instantly in speech, or writing, or in listening to the speech of other people.

Below this is the unconscious mind, in which Freud located his 'id'. Nobody, by any mental effort, can get to be aware of it in him or her. Even the most insightful psychiatrist, aided by the full goodwill and cooperation of that other person, cannot find out much about what that unconscious mind is thinking, or what it contains. I speculate that this inability extends into its connection, if any, with the unknown world.

Among the cures of psychiatry are those of disorders called 'functional' or 'hysterical' by medical doctors. An example might be a 'functional paralysis'. The patient is not malingering or trying to trick the doctor; to him or her it is a real inability. Yet it comes not from any bodily failure, but from the unconscious mind. An important clue is that it does not fit the known facts of anatomy. For example, the patient may complain of a paralyzed hand; yet the affected region does not correspond with the sort of trouble that an inactive muscle or nerve in the arm might cause. Instead, it fits the illusory anatomical notions of the patient. It can often be cured by an impressive ritual which the doctor knows is just a 'placebo', affecting the unconscious mind. Many hysterical paralyses of World War 1, which seem to been caused by 'shell shock' (as it was then known), were cured in this way.

Another psychiatric theory involving the unconscious mind is that of 'repressed memory'. Indeed, Kenneth Tynan once remarked that a neurosis is a secret you don't know you're keeping. Many mental afflictions can be alleviated by bringing 'repressed' memories or desires 'upstairs' from that mind into the conscious one. One way of doing this was to interpret the patient's sleep-dreams—indeed, Freud wrote a book about this art. (I discuss dreaming in Chapter 10). Freud reckoned that a dream was often a distorted and disguised message from the unconscious. He felt that a dream typically displayed a 'manifest content', which is what it seemed to be about. Beneath this was a 'latent content' showing what it was actually about.

It puzzles me that the unconscious mind should be such an effective censor. I can understand that it may be very remote from consciousness; indeed, the notion that it may be partly in the unknown world and not in the brain at all helps to explain why we cannot easily get at it. My notion, which is shared by many others, is that the unconscious mind holds inadmissible truths, so that much 'personal political information' is 'repressed' into it. A repressed memory can contain a vast amount of information. One psychiatrist noted that the recovered material of one repressed memory even extended to remembering the patterns on the wallpaper in the room in which the repressed event took place.

Very often a repressed memory is of some vivid event that you would expect to be retained in great detail. Furthermore, I imagine that the data must be in the conscious mind until it is 'repressed'. Has anybody investigated the process of suppression? Does it happen instantly, or within a week, or a year? Existing claims seem neither to explain how repression comes about nor why psychiatrists can so often help a patient by bringing unconscious material up. If the unconscious mind did not go in for repression in the first place, followed by censorship and distortion to keep that repression down, they would not get mentally ill. I am surprised that the organism seems to prefer continual illness to the momentary annoyance of recalling an unpleasant event. I also feel that the theory often aids dishonest claims, in the same sort of way that attractive compensation encourages people to demand recompense for doubtful ailments. Unscrupulous psychiatrists have often claimed to have uncovered all sorts of repressed memories of (for example) child abuse. Adults have frequently been made to look guilty by such testimony, and there seems not to be a good defence against it.

Psychiatric study, of course, has largely been concentrated on people who admit they are ill. I do not know of any study of simple deviants—for example, 'star guessers' who can guess better than chance. Probably the greatest deviation from the mental norm has been shown by those who founded the major religions—people such as Jesus of Nazareth, Mohammed, and Gautama Buddha. I cannot imagine their mental life, or any source for their 'enlightenment'. The religions they founded now have millions of followers, but nobody understands the way they saw the world, or the form of their enlightenments. Aldous Huxley has looked at several personal enlightenments from the outside. Like everyone else, he has to depend on whatever has been written down, but he divides such insights into two basic categories. In the 'oceanic' form of enlightenment, the universe is accepted in its totality. The subject ceases to worry about the difference between good and evil, or indeed about differences generally. There is also a more commanding 'volcanic' form of enlightenment, in which some more specific thought or action is central. Huxley's analysis reminds me of the psychiatrist Stanislav Grof,[14] who felt that we all remember the experience of being in the womb. 'Oceanic' enlightenment (Freud also used the term) relates to being safe, confined but nurtured; 'volcanic' enlightenment to being born. Both, of course, are derived from early memories. We all have such memories; it is not obvious to me why they occasionally expand into forms of 'enlightenment', if they do.

The effect of drugs on the mind

I suggest that many so-called psychedelic drugs affect the connection between the conscious mind and the unconscious one, and so may offer a clue to one or both minds. In the early days of lysergic acid diethylamide (LSD), many psychiatrists hoped that it was a useful way of mimicking schizophrenia. It could help them to understand and perhaps cure that mental disorder. The compound is an extremely powerful disturber of normal mental function. Indeed the ergot alkaloids (to which it is chemically very similar) have been implicated in many outbreaks of mental abnormality. LSD turned out not to be a useful medical model for schizophrenia. Even so, it was still valued for its ability to stir up and bring to consciousness aspects of the unconscious mind. Used in a controlled way and in a clinical setting, it played a part in restoring many mental patients to effective functioning.

Now the mere existence of biochemicals which alter the mind seems against my notion that the mind has a non-physical part. Yet many drugs, from anaesthetics onwards, owe their whole value to their mental effect. And sadly, LSD fell into the hands of criminal drug dealers. It was sold to addicts in a completely uncontrolled and unclinical way, as a trick for affecting their minds. It became an illegal substance, denied even to psychiatrists.

I continue to feel that drugs such as LSD could be informative. They might help to reveal something of what is in the unconscious mind—knowledge which, of course, might modify or even destroy my speculations. However, I am merely suggesting here that the unconscious mind may have access to data held in the unknown world. If some of that data gets transferred to the material brain for processing, LSD or drugs like it might affect the process, and influence its mental outcome. Accordingly, such 'psychedelic' drugs interest me.

Stanislav Grof has used LSD extensively. Indeed, 'oceanic' and 'volcanic' are his words: they describe aspects of the memory of intrauterine life and of being born, and connect his theories with the studies of Aldous Huxley. It seems sad to me that by outlawing LSD, we have lost one of the few ways of getting at parts of the unconscious mind. Other psychedelic drugs, notably psilocybin, the chief active principle of the Mexican mushroom used by Mexican Indian shamans, have been tried by volunteers. It seems to have had a powerful theological impact. Those volunteers were students invited to attend a Christian Good Friday service under its influence. Many of them reported strong out-of-body sensations, and strong feelings of extrasensory perception. My guess is that the psilocybin combined with the ceremony of the service to activate normally quiescent elements of the unconscious minds of the volunteers.

Telepathy

Telepathy is the direct transmission of knowledge from one living brain to another (the word was coined by Myers himself). It sometimes happens entirely at random; it generally occurs between people who are very close to each other (like brother and sister, or husband and wife). In numerous cases, someone in an emotional crisis can even induce the hallucination of his or her presence to a relative at a distance. Nearly all telepathic events seem to deal with urgent emotional matters such as birth, death, or sudden illness. Spontaneous human telepathy has been noted throughout history, and many cases have been amassed in a book of 1886, *Phantasms of the Living* by Gurney, Myers, and Podmore.[15] Many of the examples which that book quotes appear to be ones of optical images. They might fit better in that section of Chapter 10 which discusses such images; I put them here because they seem to be examples of communication between living minds. Examples have continued to occur since; indeed the great computer pioneer Alan Turing took telepathy seriously in his famous paper on machine intelligence.[35]

Telepathy used to be called 'sympathy' (which means 'thinking together'). In the 1600s Sir Kenelm Digby even implied it in claims for his sympathetic-magic powder 'weapon-salve'. This 'powder of sympathy' (which seems to have been a form of cupric sulfate) was a remedy which, if applied to a weapon, helped to heal a wound made with it—even if the wounded person was many miles away. Like other supposedly curative medicines, it hurt the injured party in the process of healing the wound. This scheme may have begun as an idea of Paracelsus, and was perhaps developed further by Gockel the younger. Digby expounded it as a fairly detailed proposition in a lecture, as a possible way of solving the problem of determining the exact time at sea: which was then very important and very difficult.

The scheme was to injure a dog and carry it on the ship, but keep the bandage of the wound on shore. At a precise time on the shore, a time-keeper would dip the bandage in the 'powder of sympathy'. This would hurt the dog on the distant ship. It would yelp in pain, telling the ship's captain the exact shore time.

Time at sea was ultimately established by Harrison's chronometer and its successors, which were very accurate clocks that work on board a ship. 'Powder of sympathy' got nowhere. However, this style of telepathy proposed to transmit a very limited amount of information—a time. I have read that a similar form of telepathy, again transmitting a single bit of information, has been tried in the Russian navy. That navy has tried it on another current hard technical problem, that of communicating with a submerged submarine. You let a mother rabbit have babies, and carry the baby rabbits on the submarine. When a submarine officer kills a baby rabbit, its mother reacts telepathically on shore—electrodes in its brain detect its dismay. This is a remarkable claim, but not absurd. American marine experts later denied that any of their submarines has made contact with its base by telepathy, though I imagine that they must have tried it out. The book *Phantasms of the Living* records many instances of dying people conveying a hallucination to a relative at a distance. Maybe a dying brain, even one of a rabbit, can act as a telepathic transmitter?

Telepathy as recorded by humans seems to be most common between those who are already emotionally close—brother and sister, husband and wife, and so on. I am intrigued by reports of Russian work claiming that telepathy can be transmitted over many hundreds of kilometres, and between particular adepts who, while they are friends and mutually aware subjects, are not intimately connected. Their contact does not last long and little information can be conveyed. Their skill is most unusual, but telepathy generally seems to convey very little information. Thus I have spoken with a person who can be deeply affected by a telepathic message that somebody has died. But my informant has no idea who has died! It might be a close relative, about whom extreme and prolonged grief would be appropriate, or it might be a casual acquaintance whose death, while regrettable, would not be a cause for extended sorrow. The dying brain may send out some sort of telepathic signal about its approaching death, but this may not include a statement of its identity. The book *Phantasms of the Living* seems to support this idea, and so do those submarine Russian baby rabbits. Another example of telepathy that has come my way is that of a mother who felt strong labour pains when her daughter many kilometers away was giving birth. Again, only one simple item of information was conveyed. I have also read of a child who knew when her father was coming home drunk and violent, and had learned to hide herself and her small sister away from the trouble to come. Again this may have been telepathy; again it implies that the transmission of a very small item of information. In the only case I know in which some subject, facing immediate death, sent a lot of detailed information to a recipient, that information was not relayed by any sort of instantaneous telepathic awareness, but by the laborious process of 'automatic writing' (Chapter 16).

Several attempts have been made to include telepathy among the normal human powers. Thus I have read that we do not know what is going on in anyone else's mind for the same reason that we don't know what is going on in our own unconscious mind: we don't want to know. I think this is obviously silly—of course we'd love to know what someone else is thinking. It would give us tremendous power, and is one of the ambitions of the ghastly dictatorship described in George Orwell's *1984*. And all of us have reserve powers which we seldom use. (I once lifted about 200 kg in a motor accident.) It is at least worth wondering if telepathy could be a natural animal gift, now (like our sense of smell) very rarely used in civilized humans. Some anthropologists have claimed that certain primitive people, strangers to technical methods of communication such as the telephone and the radio, can sometimes send messages to each other by telepathy. Again, these seem to be very simple bits of information.

The bold biological theorist Rupert Sheldrake has proposed that telepathy is indeed a natural biological power, and a pet animal may be more telepathic than its owner. Thus a dog may sense by telepathy that its master is coming home, and run in advance to the door so as to greet him. This greeting is part of the contract between the dog and its owner. I like the idea that pet and owner have a sort of contract, with rights and duties on both sides. Many anecdotes recount how domestic animals have successfully followed human owners who have moved long distances, and have finally tracked them down. Animal telepathic skill may be a factor in this achievement. In the same sort of way, witches and wizards have sometimes been accused of having 'familiars', animals with which they had an unnaturally close connection. I can imagine that they might indeed have generated or exploited a telepathic link. Discussions I have had with biologists have greatly discounted the idea of animal telepathy. If it could be built up by genetic evolution, it would be so advantageous that almost all species would show it strongly. An antelope might be very alert to the telepathic interest of a nearby lion, for example. The lion might respond with a telepathic message of its own, perhaps 'I'm not here'. The interactions of predators with prey, as well as the social styles of herd animals and human beings, would all be very different to what is observed.

This sort of argument strengthens my feeling that telepathy, if it exists, is not genetically transmitted. As so often, where facts fail to inspire me I seek ideas from fiction. Wyndham's science fiction story 'The Chrysalids' (1955) is about telepathists.[39] Nuclear radiation can induce 'mutations' of the human genome and thus alter our genetic character, usually for the worse (which is why long-lived radiation is one of the most feared hazards of nuclear war). Wyndham imagines a human society which has grown up after such a war, and is very alert to identify and prevent the spread of unusual mutations. This does not prevent a new mutation from developing– one for telepathy. In the story, a group of people discover that they have it, and for sheer survival have to conceal it from the others. Then a child shows it to an enormous extent. She is able to make contact with a distant society which accepts telepathy and which is able to rescue the threatened telepaths. At this point, Wyndham departs from our knowledge of telepathy. He assumes that telepathic power is limited by distance, so that only that one extreme mutant can make contact with the remote society, and implies that a telepathic signal indicates the direction from it comes.

In reality, as opposed to Wyndham's fiction, telepathy does not give the impression of being a genetic trait. Like many other psychic abilities, it appears rarely and randomly. It seems not to depend on distance, nor does it indicate any direction. It also seems not to run in families and has no specific position on the genome. My general feeling is that telepathy in human beings is an ability which (like an acute sense of smell) is part of human nature, but widely and shallowly distributed. It is often perceptible in primitive people, but is strongly discriminated against in a technical civilization such as ours. It operates almost only in human crises, and then only between people who are emotionally close. Hence that apparent genetic link.

If the alleged telepaths could see or hear each other, then even if nobody were deliberately cheating, information might flow unknowingly and unconsciously between them. The alleged telepaths would in fact be operating much the same trick as the horse 'Clever Hans', who detected tiny unconscious signals transmitted by his master, and the parrot Geier, who baffled the leading ethnologist Konrad Lorenz by knowing when a visitor was about to leave. Gilbert Murray the noted classicist recorded some interesting 'telepathic' experiments like this. He was frequently able to tell a lot about a topic which other people had chosen in secret, and had written about. I fear that he regarded his telepathic games as a sort of parlour trick and made no careful tests to exclude such explanations as acoustic hypersensitivity, or the reception of unwitting microsignals. So I tend to dismiss Murray's stories as a good example of an experience which, in view of its informality and lack of controls, deserves to be dismissed as an anecdote.

When radio communication was invented, a purely physical explanation seemed possible. Telepathy was radio by the brain! This idea immediately suggested experiments to determine the intensity of the signal, its speed (which should be that of a radio wave), and the exact tuning frequency which would allow it to be picked up by one brain but not another. Such experiments failed. The brain-radio theory seems to have been demolished by three separate sorts of test. First, telepathic messages seem to be immune to any sort of electromagnetic screening, even a Faraday cage that should short out a radio signal. Second, no radio apparatus can pick up human telepathic messages. In electroencephalography, electrodes are placed in close contact with the skull, when various electrical brain rhythms can be detected; these are often informatively modulated by data entering the brain. This technique indeed shows that the brain generates electrical impulses, but such signals do not seem to get out of it, nor does the brain seem able to detect electromagnetic signals beamed at it from outside. Third, telepathic messages do not obey the 'inverse square law' which governs every physical form of radiation and makes close signals much stronger than those from a distance. In fact, distance does not seem to matter; a telepathic message is not stronger or more convincing to someone nearby than it is to someone hundred of kilometres away.

My own guess is that telepathy does indeed exist, but depends on the unconscious mind. Somehow that mind is able to release a signal into the unknown world, or perhaps the information in the signal is everywhere anyway, and is available to any unconscious mind that can access it. At any rate, it is immune to the laws that govern physical-world transmission. If it is somehow accepted by the unconscious mind of the receiver, it may then be passed up to his or her conscious mind. The effect is most apparent when sender and receiver are emotionally close, but nobody understands the details. They do not seem to be genetic.

In one curious case, a seeming communication from a dead person may have in fact been a telepathic message from a living one. In 1919 Canon Douglas reported a conversation via an amateur medium with his chauffeur Réallier, who had joined the French Army in 1914, and who Douglas thought was now dead. To prove his identity, the seemingly discarnate Réallier gave many convincing details of events in his own life—events of which Douglas knew nothing, but was able afterwards to confirm completely. However, it later transpired that Réallier was not dead at all! What the amateur medium had taken to be a communication from a dead man was in fact a form of telepathy from a living one.

Another related case concerns Samuel Soal, known for his claims that the 'star guesser' Basil Shackleton could guess cards a few seconds into the future (Chapter 14).

Soal had been impressed by the powers of the medium Mrs Blanche Cooper, and devised a cunning test. He invented an imaginary person, John Ferguson, whom he concealed from Mrs Cooper, but about whom he invented several private incidents in his own mind. In some later mediumistic exchanges, Mrs Cooper talked of John Ferguson as a discarnate communicator. This suggests to me that, knowingly or unknowingly, she was somehow 'reading' the contents of Soal's mind, and took the imaginary Ferguson as having an identity of his own. Interestingly, these examples seem to have been acquired as verbal insights by the mediums concerned, and transmitted as verbal messages. They escape the implication that a telepathic message is either a single bit of information or some sort of visual image.

Anyway, I suspect that telepathy does occur. It seems to be part of an awareness of a mental world outside our diving bell. We may get information from it, while not knowing or misunderstanding where that information is coming from. If it comes from someone living through a crisis, the event is telepathy; if it comes from someone dead, it is a discarnate message. If the apparent transmitter is in the process of dying (many cases of which were described in the 1886 book *Phantasms of the Living*), I cannot usefully classify it.

Card guessing and other forms of psychic guessing

Many experiments have essentially asked subjects to guess a sequence of cards which they have been dealt. The cards are always dealt face-down, so that the subject has to make a guess every time. Most people are chance bound, and statistical analysis of their performance merely shows that their guesses are quite random. Occasionally they guess a card correctly, but this is a chance event.

Some people, maybe only one in every hundred or even fewer, are by contrast 'star guessers' (as I call them). They can guess consistently better than chance. Most of this work has been done in the Duke University paranormal laboratory in North Carolina, USA. Many publications about such games were published in the 1930s by its famous director Joseph Rhine. He soon found that standard playing cards were not ideal for this work, and asked the designer Karl Zener to develop better ones.

Even with Rhine's cleverest card-guessing games, and with the most carefully crafted Zener cards, the finest 'star guesser' would probably guess wrong most of the time. As the parapsychologist James Carpenter has dolefully said,[7] 'if the world had been constructed with the parapsychologist's convenience in mind . . . the psychic person would correctly identify all of the targets in an ESP deck each time he tried; the non-psychic would always identify only a coincidental few'. Alas, the world is not like this, and even Rhine's star guessers made lots of mistakes. They did, however, often guess a bit better than chance (Appendix B).

Many accounts of card-guessing games have been published, as have lots of critical statistical analyses. Such analyses often pointed out methodological errors, and Rhine and his successors gradually improved their guessing experiments to prevent not only deliberate subterfuge but unconscious leaks of information from the dealer to the guesser. Many papers (I have looked at several from Rhine and Schmidt) claim triumphantly that their results have some ridiculously low likelihood of having occurring by chance, but do not give any estimate of how much better than chance their star guesser was. In Appendix B, I make a few calculations about the matter. My findings are quite modest. A typical star guesser might make an inspired correct guess on a little over 7 percent of occasions. The rest of the time he or she would guess as randomly as any chance-bound subject.

Do star guessers have any sort of 'hunch' about those correct psychic guesses? Do they somehow feel right? Many studies have been made around this question, and the answer seems to be 'no'. Each guess usually feels like any other guess, even if is a correct one, or comes from some unconscious source. Some studies seem to have shown that 'felt confidence' may sometimes correlate with success, but like so much in ESP experiments, nothing is certain. My own feeling is that, even if the unconscious mind has just pushed up true and important data, it is too canny to signal the fact.

A sequence of card guessing, even with a star guesser, is often inconsistent. It may start off dramatically well, but then shows a noted decline during a sequence of trials. Towards the end of the sequence it may recover quickly or slowly, but seldom to the full initial extent. This sort of variation suggests a psychological interpretation. In the middle of a run the guesser gets bored and his or her skill declines. Furthermore, distance seldom seemed to matter. Tests in which the guesser was in one room, while the cards were in another (which might be many miles away) did not discover anything important.

Star guessers were very rare. Most people simply guessed pretty much according to the laws of chance (which I discuss a bit in Appendix A). Helmut Schmidt entered the field in the 1960s. His first experiments used random radioactive decays (those of strontium 90, whose half-life is about 29 years). His 'star guessers' could predict these 'uncaused events' a little better than chance. They also did a little better than chance in guessing pure random numbers from a table of them. I discuss some of his findings in Appendix B. They reinforce my feeling that even the starriest guessing performance, though above chance, is still quite modest. Schmidt later developed easier and safer random-number guessing machines, his Random-Number Generator (RNG) and Random-Event Generator (REG). They also exploit quantum-mechanically unpredictable occurrences (Appendix C), but electronic ones rather than radioactive events.

Card guessing is frequently very boring for everybody. One variation is the 'ganzfeld experiment' in which the guesser is invited to describe a scene in his or her mind's eye. The sender may be elsewhere, looking at a real scene, or concentrating on a specific picture intently. Either way, the sender is trying to transmit the image to the guesser. That guesser's eyes are covered with shaped half-ping-pong balls to give a featureless white visual scene, and his or her ears are saturated by headphones fed with featureless hissy 'white noise' from an electronic generator. Again, distance between the sender and the guess does not seem to matter, and the results (while very hard to score) often seem more convincing that those of card guessing. Even so, mood matters. As with card-guessing, the guesser seems less successful if he or she is bored or depressed, and his or her skill often declines steadily during the course of the trials, but may improve towards the end of a session.

Guessing better than chance: blindsight

The phenomenon of guessing better than chance does not only occur in parapsychological experiments. It is also known in an effect called 'blindsight'. This is a disorder of part of the brain concerned with vision. The victim's eyes and optical system seem in good order; nonetheless a large region of the visual scene is missing, and is replaced by a blank 'scotoma'. The victim claims to see nothing whatever in this region. If objects are placed in it, he or she asserts that they are simply not visible. And yet, asked to guess about the contents of this area, the victim does much better than chance. In some way, the 'blindseer' knows something about the visual nature of the objects in the scotoma, although this awareness is blocked from conscious visual sensation. I am reminded of optical conversion disorder, in which optical information reaching the eyes is also prevented by some mental process from going further to reach conscious awareness. (It used to be called 'hysterical blindness'.) Some stroke victims seem only aware of one side of their visual field. If asked to draw a clock face, for example, such a victim will neglect the right or left half. On one occasion a doctor used television technology to present the patient with her neglected field of view, fitting it on the side she could see. She was greatly distressed and demanded that it be removed. This makes me feel that optical neglect is at least partly an emotional phenomenon, perhaps mediated by that emotional entity, the unconscious mind. Hysterical blindness sometimes allows a limited subset of optical information to reach and influence the organism. A good fictional example occurs in the rock opera *Tommy*, a collection of songs written by the pop group The Who. The child Tommy has been badly treated by the adults in his life, and has become hysterically deaf, dumb and blind. A singer is amazed at how well he plays the extremely visual machine-game of pinball: 'This deaf, dumb, blind kid sure plays a mean pinball.'

I suspect that a similar sort of mental-hiding mechanism operates in a star guesser. The star guesser knows something about the visual content of each card, but this knowledge does not 'get upstairs' to consciousness. The 'better than chance' guesses of a star guesser may thus be promptings from the unconscious mind.

9

Observed Effects of the Unconscious Mind and the Unknown World. 2: Mechanical Effects

THE MOST INTERESTING PHENOMENON HERE is the 'poltergeist'. The word is German and means 'noisy ghost'. Such ghosts are typically active in a household setting; they may cause domestic objects such as bottles to move along a shelf, fall off it and break. Their activities are generally unseen, but sometimes a witness will see a bottle or an ornament in motion, or observe an item of cutlery being thrown. Such a thrown object may appear not to travel in the usual gravitational parabola, but to move in flight as if some force were being exerted on it during its travel. Interestingly, such a thrown object may sometimes hit a human being, but even if it seems to have been going fast, it seldom hurts the target or causes injury. As their name implies, poltergeists often make

Why Are We Conscious? A Scientist's Take on Consciousness and Extrasensory Perception
David E. H. Jones

ISBN 978-981-4774-32-1 (Hardcover), 978-1-315-16688-9 (eBook)
www.panstanford.com

noises (I have discussed acoustic effect in Chapter 11). It is also often possible to 'converse' with a poltergeist, using a code based on 'raps'. The human makes them by hitting something; the poltergeist somehow makes 'raps' in response. My musings about the deceitfulness of the unconscious mind seem reinforced by the sad fact that a poltergeist often lies.

Poltergeist action is almost entirely destructive: yet it seems more of a prank than an attempt at serious demolition. Poltergeists do not seem to undertake large physical activities such as destroying skyscrapers or locomotives or industrial cranes. Indeed, their energy seems to be roughly limited by human power. Hence, perhaps, the old joke: 'Messrs Polter, Geist and Polter will move your furniture for you.' It interests me that many poltergeists seem 'personal'. Unlike a conventional ghost (which seems bound by a particular locality, so that it may haunt a building), a poltergeist is active around a specific person, its 'focus'. That human focus may even show signs of exhaustion from its antics, suggesting that he or she is the source of its physical energy. Poltergeist action may even follow that person around, if he (or more usually she) is sent away. The poltergeist may not merely concentrate on a human focus; it may even restrict its actions to special objects, such as bottles or stones.

I was once told of a poltergeist which seemed to have entered a locked room in a church, where it had thrown the hymn books and vestments around into a wild mess. It took hours to return that room to any sort of order. And yet I feel that the seeming messy pranks of poltergeists are not evidence of their malevolence, annoyance, or jokiness, but simply of their clumsiness. My notion is that a poltergeist, as a non-material entity, simply has no experience of the physical world. I once read of one which unscrewed a bottle cap to spill the contents of the bottle, and this seems to me to show about the limiting dexterity which one might expect from an unguided poltergeist. I have never read of a poltergeist which has opened a tin to spill its contents or has contrived to open a bottle with a crimped cap. Even a young human baby takes years to acquire a sound physical sense of how to move things without breaking them, use tools to advantage, or to develop the impressive manual skills of the adult craftsman. By contrast, and as an example of learned human skill, I was once greatly impressed by a craftsman who set out to define a 90° angle on an angle-meter by eye, and got it to 89.5°. (My best was 87°.) He once sharpened a half-inch drill for me on a grinding wheel, using hand and eye alone, and got one flute two thousandths of an inch ahead of the other!

My feeling is that a poltergeist does indeed use some sort of 'psychokinetic force', but for effective action (as opposed to just making a mess) it has to express some sort of human desire—possibly an unconscious one. Thus the schoolboy Matthew Manning, who seems to have had some remarkable psychic powers, was once challenged by his young brother and sister while the whole family was at lunch downstairs. They asked him to do something poltergeisty in their upstairs bedrooms. He was still at table when they asked him to move a bedroom wardrobe and turn over a bed upstairs, and without moving from his chair, he soon announced that he had done so. After lunch, the family went upstairs to look: and indeed he had! Furthermore, he did not seem exhausted by his achievement—which contradicts my suggestion above that a poltergeist exploits the biological energy of its focus.

This story is typical of many examples of poltergeist action, though less messy than most. I have read of many mechanical changes which poltergeists seem to have made: moving things, transporting things, and so on.

Yet I have never read of any size change. Distances seem to retain their values. If something once fits something else, it always fits. My interpretation of the effect is that in some way an entity in the unknown world can take an unconscious desire from its 'focus', perhaps one about specific types of object, and turn it into a physical effect in the real world.

What is the noise of the 'noisy ghost'? I discuss that interesting question in Chapter 11, under 'acoustic effects'. I note here that the typical noise made by a poltergeist is the 'rap', a short pulse of sound rather like that made by hitting a sheet of wood with a hard striker. Acoustics is, of course, an aspect of mechanical force, but in this chapter I am concerned mainly with other types of force.

Thus an eminent scientist of the 1800s, William Crookes (who was greatly interested in allegedly psychic phenomena) once devised a balance which the noted medium Daniel Dunglas Home could attempt to influence purely by thought. One measurement showed a weight of about 6 lb—over 30 million times more than the 0.1 milligram by which I have failed to move a chemical balance by mental effort. I assume that, unlike the chaotic force often released by a poltergeist, the one exerted by Home was well directed into the equipment operated by Crookes.

Some further interesting tests were carried out in 1928 by the Danish scientist Professor Christian Winther of Copenhagen on the medium Anna Rasmussen. She was able to move a sensitive balance, and could make a pendulum swing without affecting another one nearby. However, when the apparatus was held rigid by a concrete pillar constructed in the cellar beneath it, she was unable to move either pendulum. Her purported spirit control 'Dr Lasaruz' attributed this failure to the dampness of the cellar. (I mention 'spirit controls' in Chapter 14.) This makes no sense to me—I cannot imagine why a damp cellar should be physically different from a dry one. The story makes me fear that Ms Rasmussen was playing some sort of trick on Dr Winther.

An intriguing film from Russia shows a Russian woman, Nelya Mikhailova (a pseudonym to protect her from crank interest: her real name is Nina Kulagina). She is apparently able to move objects without touching them. In the laboratory she has been able to exert a force exceeding 10 grams (100 millinewtons) on a balance, and her psychokinetic powers seem to fog undeveloped film near the objects she moves. It intrigues me that distant film seemed unaffected; indeed a successful cinematographic film was made of her activities in 1968. I do not know if the fogging effect obeyed the normal 'inverse square' of distance, or depended on some sort of screening. I am reminded that the 'paranormal inhibition' which has dogged some researchers (Chapter 6) also seems limited by distance in some way.

In the film, Nina gave a demonstration in which, in front of witnesses, journalists and photographers, she seemed able to move objects such as matches and cigarettes across a table, despite the fact that they were screened from her by a perspex shroud. Objects behind the shroud which she chose not to move remained selectively stationary. Later she separated the yolk of an egg from its white without touching it. The effects cost her a lot of physical effort. Her electroencephalogram brain record showed great excitement; her heart-beat rose to about four times its normal value; she lost about two pounds in weight over the hour or so of testing.

This story raises a question to which I have no answer: where does the energy come from for such effects? The question may be a scientific mistake. I have mused that it may come from the unknown world, and the laws of thermodynamics (which state that energy is always conserved, so that if it appears it must have come from somewhere) may not apply to transfers between the unknown world and the physical one. The Toronto group (Chapter 6) found that during a time when infection had depleted the group, so that the assembly was reduced to four and some of these felt unwell, their invented 'ghost' Philip made raps and table movements which were relatively feeble. This supports my guess that in some way the group had made contact with an element of the unknown world that was purely inorganic and had no mental aspects. Philip's energy seemed to come from his human creators—possibly from their brains (the brain takes about half the energy of the whole body). This guess also fits the notion that a poltergeist draws its energy from its human environment. The mighty efforts exerted by Mme Kulagina seem to imply that only a very small amount of her biological power was actually used to generate the 'psychokinetic energy' needed by object moving.

It sometimes happens that much depends on a mechanical event that may possibly be influenced by psychokinetic forces. A good example is the rolling of dice. Many games use rolling dice essentially as random-number generators. If dice can be influenced by 'psychokinetic' forces, they are more likely to roll the way the psychokinetically able player wants.

Many experiments on rolling dice were conducted in the famous laboratory (Chapter 6) established at Duke University in North Carolina and headed by Joseph Rhine. He found that as with card-guessing games (Chapter 8), a few of his 'star guessers' seemed to throw dice significantly better than chance. He tried various ways of casting the dice, both in the traditional way by throwing from a cup and by a range of mechanical devices, but none seemed to have a dramatic effect on the random nature of the throw. One obvious question is, what force (in newtons, say) is deployed by a good psychokineticist? The Swedish engineer Forwald looked at this in many ways. He varied the weight, size, surface nature, and number of his dice, and the sort of surface they were thrown onto. His results were by no means precise, but he seems to have found that for beechwood dice weighing two grams each, a typical psychokinetic force might be about 3 millinewtons, or 0.3 grams weight. This might not make much difference to a rolled dice.

My feeling is that honest dice are pretty good random-number generators. They may be slightly affected by hard psychokinetic wishing, but any such effect is probably largely cancelled out by the other wishers also playing the game. Even one of Rhine's 'star guessers' would probably not do dramatically better against mere chance-bound players. There are, of course, bent games, in which some trickster has 'loaded' the dice. But only a very unwary gambler would get into a craps game as bent as the one envisaged in Damon Runyon's story 'Broadway Financier', in which Big Nig expounds the art of sneaking in two loaded dice: 'switching in a pair of tops' in the jargon.

A related study of a possible psychokinetic force was again set up in the Duke University paranormal laboratory. It did not use dice, but steel balls. About 1200 such balls were released in a special randomizer, so as to fall into a receiving 32-channel chute. In the absence of any observer, they spread out in the chute in the normal, expected, 'Gaussian' distribution. Hard mental willing by an observer seemed to be able to make the balls deviate detectably from the distribution; even so, the results seemed not to give any sense of the mode of action or the strength of the psychokinetic force felt by the balls.

Large psychic forces, equivalent to many newtons and many kilograms of weight, have often been reported. Thus the alleged levitation of some holy people occurs in much old religious literature. Similarly, large 'psychic forces' were often apparently deployed and reported in Victorian séances. The turning of heavy tables and even their levitation were investigated by scientists of the highest repute, including Michael Faraday, Madame Curie, Lord Rayleigh, and Sir William Crookes. In 1927 Crookes himself told his colleague Sir William Bennett that 'on that very hearth rug where you are standing' he had seen Daniel Dunglas Home levitate himself.

Levitation has even been alleged to occur in the modern world. It is a trick supposedly demonstrated by some Eastern sages. Thus in a poem, T. S. Eliot saluted his criminal cat Macavity, whose 'powers of levitation would make a fakir stare'. Though fictional, this poem acknowledges claims which have often been made about strange powers in the mystic East. Thus Maharishi Mahesh Yogi promoted his ideas by setting up a number of establishments around the world. Among other notions, they disseminated his claim for levitation through deep meditation, a practice he called 'Vedic flying'. His foundation at Mentmore Towers in Buckinghamshire became known among locals as 'the third London airport'. I am sceptical, and not only because no photographs were allowed. One disillusioned disciple described Vedic flying as 'bouncing on your bum'.

I suspect that a lot of such displays were self-delusion and trickery. A Victorian séance was often set up in dim lighting or even total darkness. It was often under the control of a special 'medium' who sat in a 'cabinet' across which a curtain could be drawn, thus concealing his or her activities. The alleged psychic forces thus created might have satisfied a gullible audience. I have read of at least one account of a levitation fraud being brought about by a lifting rope. An interesting test was once conducted by Dr William Jackson Crawford, a Victorian lecturer in engineering at Belfast University. He arranged for the chair of the medium (Miss Kathleen Goligher, later Mrs S. G. Donaldson) to be mounted in a weighing scale. When she levitated a table, he noted that the weight registered by the scale increased by the weight of the table. She seems to have been holding it up in some way. Later Crawford wrote a book[9] in which he commented of a séance that the 'usual table-rappings and levitations occurred and were ascribed of course to spirit operations'. I have to be suspicious. The Toronto inventors of the fictitious ghost Philip tried to get him to levitate a table and may once have succeeded for a short time. So perhaps forces from the unknown world can sometimes be of sufficient intensity to levitate heavy objects. However, such forces are very rare. Engineers never have to bother with them. 'Paranormal levitation' was commonly reported in Victorian séances, but I am not convinced that it was a real effect.

Respected scientists have claimed to witness it in the past. Nonetheless, while many cases of small forces have been reported, I am suspicious of the claims made for this big one. It happens that we know a lot about genuine levitation from the experiences of the aeronautical engineers who worked on the 'flying bedstead' experimental aerial vehicle. This was levitated by the thrust of a downward-pointing jet engine, and ran into a lot of trouble.

Consider the problem. If you apply the right amount of upward force to (say) a table, it will float in the air. Too little force and it will not move at all; too much and it will accelerate upwards and hit the ceiling. If your force is not applied precisely through the centre of gravity of the table, it will tilt violently. If your force is not exactly vertical, its sideways component will push the table sideways till it hits a wall. To bring it down safely, the force must be reduced by a small amount so controllably that the table is not damaged by too rapid a descent. Accordingly, a successful levitation needs continuous control: either by the person being levitated or (in the case of a demonstration in a séance) by the medium in secret charge of either an unknown force or a fraudulent operation. It interests me that no report of 'paranormal levitation' seems to have encountered these side-effects.

Psychokinetic 'energy'

In this discussion of mechanical effects, I have largely avoided talking about the source of energy used by (for example) poltergeists. Yet as a physical scientist, I am strongly aware of the law of conservation of energy. Energy can't just appear: it has to come from somewhere. But where? It may come from the human beings who set up or witness the phenomena, or it may be supplied from the unknown world.

The Toronto group (Chapter 6) found that their invented ghost, 'Philip', was able to move their table around, but only once did they record a brief levitation (which I mention above). Even so, they felt that they had activated some unknown force and often claimed to have produced 'psychokinesis by committee'. Like many other workers, they felt that the psychokinetic force they had observed might, if tamed and technically handled, transform several fields—particularly those of aiding the disabled and infirm. My assumption here is that the force, and the energy implied by its movement, comes in some way from the unknown world. That force seems to be capable of disturbing balances, setting pendulums swinging, making raps, and even lifting tables. Yet it is not at all obvious how it works. One of the most interesting reports of the Toronto workers was that it could make their wooden table move, apparently by exerting some force on its leg joints. The furniture designer had intended those joints to be rigid, and indeed they always were as long as the table functioned as a normal piece of inert furniture. Yet under the influence of the fictitious Philip they became not only flexible but energetically active—in much the same way that a human muscle not only changes shape, but exerts a lot of force in the process, and consumes biological energy while it does so. Furthermore, this energetic flexing of normally rigid joints was not chaotic or random: it was organized in such a way that the table could walk, dance, and even climb. The Toronto workers used several tables in the course of their research, and Philip could make any of them move. He even evoked dramatic table movements under the bright lights needed by TV and ciné cameras, so that film exists of that movement! Since Philip never existed, except in the minds of the eight people who invented him, I assume that the energy needed to cause the movements and raps shown by the table must have come either from the people in the group or from the unknown world. This suggests that the unknown world outside our diving bell can supply us with energy, and can even (if we know how to direct it properly) exert that energy in useful and exact ways for us. Accounts such as those of the Toronto group, however, make me as a physical scientist very unhappy. I would like to believe that the properties of all materials are fixed and well known, and the laws governing energy are even more so. Yet many cosmologists assert that the materials we know about constitute very little of the universe, which is largely composed of unknown dark matter and (even more unknown) dark energy. So I am prepared to tolerate the notion that the world as a whole may be far removed from one we manipulate in the laboratory and the factory.

10

Observed Effects of the Unconscious Mind and the Unknown World. 3: Optical Effects

THIS DISCUSSION HAS TO CENTRE on ghosts, for the overwhelmingly popular theory of ghosts is that each is in some way the animation of the soul of someone dead, which has come back to haunt the physical world as a visual apparition. However, the obvious counter-theory is that such effects are simply a form of hallucination. A hallucination is a malfunction of the sensory system, leading it to report something which is not there. It can disrupt any sensory system. (I myself once answered a telephone, convinced that it had been ringing. It hadn't: I had had an acoustic hallucination.) A typical medical hallucination is the illusion of feeling the creep of small creatures on the skin, a common sensory delusion is delirium tremens. It is a private feeling and cannot be

Why Are We Conscious? A Scientist's Take on Consciousness and Extrasensory Perception
David E. H. Jones

ISBN 978-981-4774-32-1 (Hardcover), 978-1-315-16688-9 (eBook)
www.panstanford.com

tested by an external carer, though that carer may note that no small creatures can be seen on the skin. There are, of course, many ways to distinguish a hallucination from a sensory reality. A simple one is permanence, or even just persistence. Instrumental tests are often useful. Some of the 'phantasms' recorded by Gurney, Myers and Podmore (Chapter 8) even showed a reflection in a mirror, or cast a visible shadow.

Accordingly, the first move in any discussion of optical effects has to be to differentiate between ghostly apparitions and simple hallucinations. I shall begin by denouncing conjuring. Many people, in Thomas Carlyle's bitter words, 'hunger and thirst to be bamboozled' and a large trade in illusioneering has grown up to satisfy them. A stage magician deliberately sets out to mislead an audience and is often very clever at directing attention away from some subtlety, or gulling the audience into going along with an ingenious fiction. The success of theatrical 'magic' depends on a fact we pretty much accept all the time. Our senses are reliable, and the brain just takes their findings as they come. Those senses exist to tell us about the surrounding physical world, and we want them be true and straight. They usually work. But the stage magician knows their weaknesses and assumptions, how to trick them, and how to set up a delusive fiction.

Occasionally, however, hallucinations seem to be inspired by the unknown world. The neurologist Benjamin Libet has found that it takes about half a second for any new sensory impression to give rise to conscious sensation. He argues that this half-second delay gives enough time for some brain process to fiddle with the sensing apparatus of the brain and allows it to make up a false report. This time delay might also allow several senses to combine, giving an 'apparition' which seems to include (for example) both sound and vision—such as a visible ghost which makes audible footsteps.

Ghost stories occur in all societies and throughout history. I feel that this genre of story is unlikely to have made it into literature without a few real examples. The oldest one I know is told by the Roman orator Pliny the Younger, who set it down in about 100 AD. He describes a haunted house in Athens, in which the philosopher Athenodorus was working when he heard rattling chains. They came from a ghost: an old man with a beard and heavy iron fetters. Athenodorus followed the ghost into the garden, where it indicated a site. Digging at this point revealed a shackled skeleton. When these remains were dug up and given proper burial rites, the haunting ceased. Athenodorus was able to carry on with his work.

Every society seems to have maintained a belief that 'ghosts' exist, and are visions of dead people: visions best avoided. Thus one traditional Scottish prayer goes: 'From ghoulies and ghosties / And long-leggedy beasties / And things that go bump in the night, / Good Lord deliver us!' One way of avoiding a ghost is by treating a dead body appropriately (as by burying it in consecrated ground). Even ancient corpses such as those of Cro-Magnon man (whose remains are estimated to be some 40,000 years old) often show modifications suggesting some sort of belief like this. Sophocles' play *Antigone* (about 440 BC) concerns the attempts of Antigone to have the body of her brother buried properly. Samuel Johnson seems to have felt that ghosts were real. In the 1700s he wrote: 'It is wonderful that five thousand years have now elapsed since the creation of the world, and still it is undecided whether or not there has ever been an instance of the spirit of any person appearing after death. All argument is against it: but all belief is for it.' William Golding has expressed his dismay at discovering an Iron Age rubbish-pit into which the body of a woman had apparently been thrown without ceremony. Aldous Huxley's novel *Brave New World* gains much of its force by imagining a society which has discarded any respect for the dead. Many towns maintain graveyards with tombstones and impede builders who want to develop the land. This universal reverence for dead people may seem irrational. It appears to imply that many people whose corpses were not properly disposed of may appear as ghosts. This worry may be particularly strong for people killed in accidents or in battle. Hence, perhaps, the way that the sites of major military disasters are often sanctified as 'war graves'. I also recall the public disquiet caused by the body snatchers or 'resurrection men' of the early 1800s, who extracted corpses from their graves to provide bodies for medical dissection. The disturbing feeling that the living can generate for the dead may even exist in animals—I have read of an elephant seen apparently grieving over the remains of a dead elephant.

A common social notion is that a ghost is in some way a relic of a person who has lived. When a human baby is born, it typically lives for about 70 years, and then dies. It may then generate a ghost. I have never heard of anyone being haunted by a human pre-relic waiting to be born. That asymmetry strikes me as odd. I have even contemplated an odder asymmetry. Let us suppose that there are many other conscious intelligent beings in the universe (this seems supported by the Anthropic Principle, which I discuss rather dismissively in Appendix E, although many science fiction writers support it, and so do many eminent scientists. Enrico Fermi's support for it is in Chapter 17). I particularly recall a TV character called ALF, for Alien Life Form. Suppose that when ALF dies, it leaves a ghost in the unknown world. If ALF came from a thriving community created by evolution, that ghost might be one of a huge number in that world. One might occasionally appear to a human observer, who would probably take it as merely a puzzling hallucination. As far I am aware, human beings only see human ghosts.

This train of thought invites a guess. How many ghosts should here be? For human ghosts the calculation is reasonably simple. If we assume that humanity is 3 million years old, having evolved from apelike creatures about that length of time ago, and that for much of that time till the near present the human population was a few million or so, then something like 10^{11} human beings have lived and died. If every dead human being has left a ghost, there should be 10^{11} ghosts, which is about 15 ghosts for every person now alive. 10^{11} is a huge number, especially if we consider that most people have never seen a ghost. By far the greatest number of those ghosts can never have appeared to anybody. Indeed, most recorded ghosts are those of dead persons known to, or at least known about by, the hauntee (a name I have invented for the observer of a ghost). Non-human ghosts, such as that of ALF and maybe of many others of the kind, evade any feasible calculation. Nobody can guess how many non-human conscious intelligent beings the universe may contain, nor for how long, nor whether such beings die, nor if so any of them leave ghostly relics.

All such entities exist (if they do) in the unknown world outside our diving bell. They make only weak and occasional contact with the physical world we know about, often by sonic signs such as footsteps or raps. Indeed sometimes such noises are the only sign of ghostly presence (I discuss acoustic effects in Chapter 11). I have never read of a case in which a ghost has affected a purely material object: as by setting off a burglar alarm, for example. It is a common notion that a ghost is in some way the relic of a person who has lived. One powerful optical example was recorded by Myers. The hauntee was an American commercial traveller, who in 1876 'saw' (in bright sunlight) an image of his dead sister. The image vanished before he could even call out her name, but he saw her so clearly that he remembered a small scratch on her face. This was later identified; it was made by accident on her corpse, shortly after her death.

A ghost is often taken as being a relic of somebody who lived at that site in the past. Thus I have read of a ghost who walked through a wall, and subsequent architectural research revealed that there had in the past been a doorway at that point. I have even read of a case where a pet dog was apparently able to react to a ghost. If we accept the idea that a ghost appears to you by acting in some way on your unconscious mind, and that you need to have such a mind to be conscious at all, this makes sense. It implies that a dog has an unconscious mind, which allows it to 'see', or at least react to, the ghost. This idea also suggests that a ghost is not always a simple individual hallucination. It may have enough reality for several people (one of whom may be a dog) to see it. However, no matter what the reality of a ghost may be, its clothes have to be entirely material and should be the same for all observers. Yet I know of at least one report in which different observers reported different clothing! I have never heard of a naked ghost, and suspect that that each observer has his or her own idea of the most appropriate clothing to imagine around it.

A ghost is often thought of as haunting a specific volume, typically an old house in which many people have died, so that there are several candidates for persons returning to haunt the site of their death. Modern buildings, in which nobody has yet died, are perhaps less fertile in ghostly terms. How much volume in the physical world might a ghost 'haunt'? If it haunted a little volume like 1 cm^3, almost no human being would notice. If it haunted a big one like 1 km^3, a human who observed the haunting would see only part of it, and might take it to be it a small local phenomenon. This 'local effect' arouses my interest. A popular notion is that of a 'haunted house' or even a 'haunted room' in a house, giving a total haunted volume of maybe 10 m^3. This implies that a typical haunted volume is about that held by or belonging to an individual human being, and indeed suggests that the ghost has some particular interest in the human being thus singled out. In a large building containing many self-contained dwellings, only one may be 'haunted'. In general, ghost hauntings seem 'place oriented', so that a haunted house often remains haunted even if its occupiers move away and new ones move in. This may not always be true; ghostly effects may depend on the human culture of the occupiers. I know of a haunted house that became a carpet factory, and later a factory for Islamic textile workers. They may have had a totally alien culture. In any case, they were not bothered by the ghost.

To continue this spatial argument, what is the size of a ghost? A mere personal hallucination may not have a size, but a real object should have one. A ghost, as the relic of a human being, must presumably project an image of about human size. *Phantasms of the Living* (Chapter 8) gives many examples of human hallucinations apparently created by telepathy and seemingly having the right sort of size. This size idea is contradicted by an intriguing fictional example. In 1820 William Blake drew a picture, now in the Tate Gallery in London, of the ghost of a flea. He drew it the size of a man. A flea had told him, he said, how at the creation it was at first intended to make him as big as a bullock, but in view of his evil nature he was made much smaller. Blake claimed later that his picture reflected the abomination of the flea, which though very small had this huge unpleasant ghost. A related fictional example comes from the cartoonist Peter Blegvad.[4] In his cartoon strip 'Leviathan', he drew the hero Levi going to hell. There he met Mr B. L. Z. Bub, the devil, who as 'Lord of the fleas' was the size of a flea himself. Blegvad might have given Blake ideas! So might Thomas Nashe, a dramatist of the late 1500s who once imagined human beings infested with tiny devils: evil bacteria we might call them today. Occasionally people have claimed to have seen human forms of smaller or larger size than normal: fairies or giants, say. I reckon these must have been some sort of hallucination, of which the human observer got the size wrong. Elves, goblins, and other humanoid creatures of which no corpses have been found, but which have occurred in stories from many societies, may also be based on similar visions. They cannot have been a misinterpretation of some real animal, or of any creature from the physical world.

Anyway, a ghost seems not be a purely personal hallucination. It can appear to several people, but not everyone can see it. Furthermore, it can even be exorcised. I suspect that a good exorcist is far out on the rim of some mental Gaussian bell (Appendix A), and may also be a potential medium or 'star guesser'. Of course, to be an effective exorcist, you have to be able to see the ghost (and I have heard of a hauntee who could not see a ghost, although the exorcist could. The hauntee was just strongly worried by some presence.) One exorcist discourages ghosts with powerful strobe lighting and violent pop music—which would dismay a lot of humans, too. One theory is that a ghost so discouraged does not vanish. It merely retreats into its non-material world and no longer appears as a visual apparition in that physical locality.

Incidentally, seeing a ghost poses a curious optical problem. If you see that ghost, you presumably do not see the scene behind it. Even if the ghost is translucent, it obscures its background somewhat, so you see that scene less clearly. If you are an ordinary viewer and do not see the ghost, you presumably 'look right through it' and see the scene behind it unattenuated. I have never seen a good photograph of a ghost; they frequently occur in dark conditions, which supports the notion that they are essentially an optical hallucination.

One interesting claim is that a ghost can cool the room in which it appears. This may not simply be a subjective human impression. Workers in the Toronto Society for Psychical Research (who created the fictitious artificial ghost Philip, and indeed hoped to obtain a visible ghostly apparition of him—Chapter 6) noted that external observers felt a 'cool breeze' flowing across a table on which their artificial ghost manifested itself. Indeed, in some paranormal experiences, thermometer falls of up to 5 degrees Celsius have been recorded. I have suggested that the cooling effect caused by a ghost derives from the fact that it comes from a very cold place.[14] This fits the notion that ghostly experiences derive from a world which is very cold. McMullen (Chapter 7) has suggested that the energy needed for poltergeist action might come from cooling the room. This idea contravenes the laws of thermodynamics—which may not apply to exchanges between the unknown and the physical worlds. But it interests me that many paranormal phenomena seem to involve cooling. A fictional example[33] occurs in Nevil Shute's *No Highway*. The eccentric scientist Mr Theodore Honey distributes recording thermographs around a house haunted by a poltergeist, to see if it has any effect on the local temperature.

Sleep-dreams

Dreams are presumably created in the unconscious mind and pushed upstairs to the sleeper. They may well have no connection with whatever is coming in through the senses of the dreamer. Accordingly, they may be a very effective way of exploiting the stillness of the mind that comes with the absence of consciousness; sleep may quieten those 'chattering monkeys' (Chapter 4). The novelist William Golding wrote that in sleep 'all the unsorted stuff comes flying out as from a dustbin upset in a high wind'. He perhaps regarded dreams as a sample of the 'unsorted stuff' in the unconscious mind. Anyway, both psychiatrists seeking clues about that mind and ordinary people looking for a way into it have taken dreams seriously. Many primitive tribes have felt that a sleeping dream results from the soul of the slumbering person waking up, looking about and wandering around. Tribal members have often been greatly perturbed by the notion of the sleeping car in a train. They fear that the sleeper may dream; his or her soul may wake up, wander around, and be unable to return to the sleeping body again because the train has moved on! If that theory were correct, a dream should consist entirely of scenes from the environment of the dreamer. It seldom does. Religious organizations have often reckoned that dreams were messages from the Gods, and have been concerned about 'divinations' of the future based on dreams. They seem to describe a future event—either one that will inevitably happen or some disaster which may be averted or minimized by informed precognitive action. Accordingly, I suspect that a dream may not be a mere personal story invented by the unconscious mind of the dreamer, which routinely warps or disguises it before sending it 'upstairs' to the dreaming mind. It may have elements which are 'outside time', inserted into it by the unknown world I am musing about. This idea is reinforced by a story recounted in Freud's famous book *The Interpretation of Dreams*. The dreamer Maury dreamed of a trial during which he was convicted of some crime during the French Revolution, and sentenced to be beheaded on the guillotine. The sentence was carried out, and Maury was woken up by the headboard of the bed falling on his neck. Either he dreamt the whole dream in an instant at that moment, and his memory projected it backwards to make sense of it, or in some way the dream was set up around the falling of the headboard, which had not yet happened. John Dunne's famous book of 1927, *An Experiment with Time*, also discusses the possible divinatory aspect of dreams. A group of people who conducted shared sessions of meditation over three years even came occasionally to have 'shared dreams'. Each member of the group recorded his or her memory of a dream and found it identical in all details with the record made by another member of the group. This seems to me to be an interesting case of unconscious telepathy (I discuss telepathy in Chapter 8).

Psychiatric interest in dreams has usually concentrated on the case in hand, which means concentrating on the present while disregarding the future. Freud's book seems to have started a huge folk industry which studies dreams in terms of the current challenges facing the dreamer. Even professional psychiatrists try to probe the unconscious mind of a patient in this way. Thus when the great physicist Wolfgang Pauli became depressed in 1932, he went to the great psychiatrist Carl Jung, who offered to study his dreams.

The notion that dreams might predict something of the future was studied in a 'dream laboratory', active during the 1970s in the Maimonides Medical Center at Brooklyn New York, USA. (Incidentally, that laboratory found that dreams seem to have the same sort of internal time that an investigator would deduce. The researchers used electroencephalography to study the brain's dream signals from outside. Their findings seem to go against the notion that Maury's dream occurred in a quick temporal flash.) The Maimonides Center developed from the work of Nathanial Kleitman, who had discovered that dreaming often leads the sleeper to make rapid-eye movements (REMs) under the closed lids of the eyes. Such movements could be detected without disturbing the sleeper, by sticking little electrodes around the eyes. When the sleeper was wakened after such electrodes had indicated REMs, he or she often reported having had a dream, and could frequently describe it in detail. Of course, you can't ask a sleeper to guess a sequence of cards, but you can ask him or her to gaze intently at a picture before going to sleep, and can ask later what any dream was about. It is also possible to have an 'agent' who stays awake and tries by mental concentration to transmit something (such as a picture the agent is looking at) to the sleeper. Yet another possibility is to expose the sleeper to (for example) a slide show, maybe even after the dreaming session. One 'star dreamer' in particular seemed able to dream precognitively, for example, about a slide show he was given a day later.

Dream research is very expensive and troublesome to set up and run. I fear that too little work has been reported to underpin any convincing analysis. We merely have a large set of anecdotes. Even so, my sense remains that the unconscious mind can indeed construct a dream which is somehow influenced or shaped by events which, in the physical world, have not yet happened.

The out-of-body experience (or OBE) and the near-death experience (or NDE)

I find these experiences hard to believe or understand, but they were recorded by Myers in the 1800s and have been reported since. The subject appears to have been freed from his or her body, and to be able to move by flying or drifting to some distant location: the apparent event has been called 'astral planing'. An OBE subject can often observe people or things at that location. Sometimes people at the site can even be aware in some way of the subject's 'presence'. Meanwhile, observers of the subject's body report that it is still there and has not moved. Myers called the acquisition of new information about a distant site 'telaesthesia'. Thus some Australian Aborigines have claimed, for example, that a certain type of whistling in the ears is a signal that your elder brother is thinking of you. The message seldom reveals where he is or what he is thinking. A more interesting claim is that some Westerners, after making the mind blank and being given a geographical location, have reported a 'remote viewing' of that location. They have claimed to see 'in their mind's eye' details of objects at the site–including seeing the inside of a building that could not be seen by an external observer. A 'remote viewer' might be extracting visual information from the mind of someone inside the building and looking at the scene: this would make the experience a form of telepathy (Chapter 8). I recall the alleged words of the dead Oscar Wilde, taken down by a medium, that he was without eyes in the spirit world, but had seen a tea plantation, in what was then Ceylon, through the eyes of a living Tamil girl. This suggests that information acquired by the physical senses of someone alive can sometimes be acquired by an entity in the unknown world. If that information were then transferred to another human mind, the outcome would be a sort of remote viewing. Alternatively, the remote viewer might be acquiring information about the distant site that was not in anybody's living mind at the time. This style of telaesthesia would then be a form of 'clairvoyance'.

The subject of an OBE experience often reports 'seeing' things on the journey to and from the site. This has to be some sort of illusion, as the eyes of the OBE subject are back with the rest of the body. The 'astral planer' would not be able to see anything with his or her eyes. Indeed, the 'thoughtographer' Ted Serios (Chapter 11) began his career with an OBE in which he decided to take a camera along with him, so as to record the site he visited, and anything interesting along the way to it. Some OBE subjects report astral-plane fantasies, such as going to distant planets, but those who restrict their journeys to testable earthly locations do indeed seem somehow to be able to acquire true information about such locations. I am not aware of any OBE subject who has reported anything not known to some human mind, so it makes sense to consider this experience to be a strangely embellished form of imaginative telepathy. A counter-example would be a report of conditions on an uninhabited island, which was only later visited and inspected to check the report.

Such claims remind me of the strange way in which many animals are able to 'find their way home', often from vast distances. They too seem able to obtain information about a distant site. Many creatures love their territory more than anything else, and Rupert Sheldrake has suggested (Chapter 8) that they may exploit telepathy—which I suggest above is a form of contact with the unknown world. I now further speculate that those puzzling feats of animal navigation may imply some other way of getting information from the unknown world, as may happen in some forms of telaesthesia, and may even occur in molecules (Chapter 11). However, many reports from this area puzzle me. I make no claims to understand them and have no guesses to account for them.

Another related experience, which I also do not understand, is the NDE, or near-death experience. One of the best-known cases is that of the aircraft pilot Douglas Bader. After a major air crash, he had the sense of going down a corridor of light to his death. Medical attention brought him back to life, and though severely crippled (he had lost his legs), he claimed thereafter to have no fear of death. Even the sceptical philosopher Sir Alfred J. Ayer has described his recollection of an NDE. He claimed that in it he could debate the laws of time and space with the government of the universe. 'On the face of it,' he later said, 'these experiences are rather strong evidence that death does not put an end to consciousness.' Another interesting example of NDE is recorded by the neurosurgeon Eben Alexander. He spent about a week in a coma brought by bacterial meningitis. Brain scans of his unconscious body revealed no detectable activity. However, he returned to consciousness with a vivid memory of having visited another world, and later wrote a book about his memories.[1] Some NDE subjects even remember the strange sensation of looking down on their own body. This cannot be real, as the eyes by which that subject claimed to see the body were still down there attached to it. It has, however, resulted in at least one practical test. An intensive-care unit has attached notices to the tops of its lampshades, so that any soul which escapes and later returns to its body can be asked what it read during its excursion. As far as I know, the intensive-care unit has not set up a system to look upwards for a ghost.

An intriguing piece of fiction by H. G. Wells,[36] 'Under the Knife', features a sort of NDE. In Wells's story, the soul of a man leaves his body during a medical operation. That soul rapidly loses contact with the Earth and finds itself in interstellar space. This makes perfect scientific sense: a soul would not be attracted by the gravity of the Earth and would not orbit the Sun. Wells did not take this clever notion to any conclusion relevant for us. But if every human being leaves a soul, and if that soul survives as an entity in the unknown space, there should be about 10^{11} human souls there by now (I estimate this huge number above). A volume of 10^{70} km^3 (the volume of physical space we can know about; Chapter 2) should give lots of room for all of them. Accordingly, ghostly souls seldom appear to us because they are all in interstellar space! Heaven indeed has many mansions. Later (1971) D. A. Wright[38] also proposed that most ghosts should be in space by now; sadly, his argument rests on flawed physics.

I have failed to make any obvious sense of remote viewing, OBE and NDE in terms of my musings about the world outside our diving bell. Such experiences fit my general view that the conscious mind, via the unconscious mind, can sometimes make contact with the unknown world. However, I also suspect that there is much coding and alteration in information which is transferred from the unknown world to the unconscious mind (Chapter 16). I also reckon that the unconscious mind disguises its notions further in the process of shifting some of them 'upstairs' to the conscious mind (which is why, as I discuss above, dreams need 'interpreting'). I recall how I developed many illusions in my own stroke. They were generally based on genuinely observed facts, but became elaborated into extremely strange fantasies. Thus I had observed, in one of my few moments of near-wakefulness, that I was in a bed. It was a standard hospital bed, with aluminium curtain rails above it and around it. In my fantasy these were part of an optical data-transmission system by which data on the ward and the people in it could be transferred to some remote bureaucratic centre where decisions were taken. I puzzled over the technology it might employ. It would be very hard to decipher my original curtain-rail observations from my wild illusions about them. Accordingly, I do not take the conscious memories of Bader and Alexander, and other such human recollections, very seriously. I suspect that such memories derive from some genuine experience or physical observation, but are very imaginative developments of it. They support my feeling that the human mind can occasionally make contact with the unknown world, but it would probably be a mistake to regard them as providing true information about its nature. I record above something of my uncertainties in this area. However, there have been several reports like this. While I can query their details, I do not wish to ignore them.

11

Observed Effects of the Unconscious Mind and the Unknown World. 4: Acoustic and Other Physical Effects

Some ghostly apparitions seem to have been accompanied by noise: footsteps, door-handle rattlings, raps. Such noises suggest some sort of impact on two different senses at once: that of sight and that of sound. They make little obvious sense: a weightless apparition should not make audible footsteps, and one that can go through a door would not have to rattle the handle. Poltergeists also produce raps. The whole social phenomenon of spiritualism developed from a rapping poltergeist in the household of Mr Fox in Rochester in the USA, in 1848.

Many raps have been recorded by sound equipment. In 1972 the Toronto Society for Psychical Research,[29] encountered rapping noises (Chapter 6) during their extraordinary experiment of 'inventing' a ghost. A group

Why Are We Conscious? A Scientist's Take on Consciousness and Extrasensory Perception
David E. H. Jones

ISBN 978-981-4774-32-1 (Hardcover), 978-1-315-16688-9 (eBook)
www.panstanford.com

of investigators in that Society set up a completely fictional character, 'Philip', and fitted him out with an equally fictitious background. He was imagined as an English nobleman of the 1600s. He played a part in the English Civil War of that time, featuring King Charles I and Oliver Cromwell. He was given a tragic domestic life, and killed himself at the age of 30 by throwing himself from the battlements of his castle. The buildings he was imagined to inhabit exist in England, but the Toronto group gave them structural elements that never existed.

The group initially had 14 people, but some members withdrew, leaving eight 'regulars'. They met every week for a year and indulged in a joint meditation about Philip. After about a year with little success, the group ultimately found that Philip could rap on the table. During such sessions, nobody in the Toronto group made any attempt to rap on the table by himself or herself. The group could even ask Philip questions by means of those raps. To simplify the exchanges, they only asked questions that could be answered by one rap for yes and two raps for no. Questions that Philip did not want to answer (such as ones about his sexual life) produced scratching noises from the table. The group did not know at that time that poltergeists sometimes also produce scratching noises. The ultimate aim of the group was to create a visible apparition of Philip, but this ambition failed. Those raps, however, seemed real and not of human origin. They were able to record many of them on sound equipment, and later had them analyzed sonically. The raps recorded by the Toronto group are scientifically well authenticated and very convincing, but other paranormal raps have also been recorded and studied sonically. They all seem to show that such raps die away faster than ones created by normal physical knocking.

The Toronto raps appear to have been originated by movements of the table surface. Thus the group often noted that a weak rap could not be heard, but could be felt by the fingers as some sort of vibration of that surface. Furthermore, the raps were usually spatially localized. Philip could produce a rap that seemed to be directed at the person who asked him a question, and often seemed to answer the question before the questioner had completed the verbal sentence. This suggests that Philip was reading the mind of the questioner, and reinforces my speculation that an entity in the unknown world may be able to 'read' an idea in a conscious mind before it gets translated into language. There might be other indications that Philip's response was personal—thus the questioner often felt that the responding rap originated under his or her fingers. Other members of the group usually heard it, but did not have the impression that it was specifically directed at them. Philip once created a joint rap that went to every member of the group. If asked, he was able to create raps which seemed to originate from a region on the plastered wall of the room, but most of his raps came from the table.

The Toronto group tried to imitate Philip's raps by knocking on their table with fingers, rings, pencils, and so on. They used several sorts of object, and indeed several tables, but never got anything to sound right. I have great respect for the subtle awarenesses and sensitivities of the human ear (which is why, in my opinion, old-fashioned vinyl recordings continue to be sold and to have value. They sound different from, and more pleasing than, modern digital recordings). Accordingly, I pay a lot of attention to the way things sound to the ear. Any sound is a pattern of movement of the molecules of the air. It travels at the speed of sound (of course) and is usually launched into the air by some sort of disturbance of a solid object—such as the cone of a loudspeaker, or our own vocal cords. A sharp pulse of sound is often called a 'rap'. It is frequently made by physically hitting a wooden sounding-board with a solid object used as a striker. A sound made in this way starts suddenly at the moment of impact and dies away relatively gradually as the vibrating board loses energy. Philip's raps were not like this. Sonic analysis revealed that his raps differed from physical ones by decaying more sharply. The finding makes me feel that during a rap the wood of the table altered its physical character. It became momentarily more flexible, easier to bend, and absorbed more energy with each movement.

Another interesting sonic effect has been claimed by Konstantin Raudive, a Latvian who lived in Germany. He has claimed that a radio tuned to the 'white noise' between stations may pick up soft extraneous voices. He even claimed to get voices from blank tape, or from the random noise generated by solid-state electronic diodes. In 1971 a major recording company used its own equipment and engineers to make an 18-minute recording under his direction. Nothing was heard during the session, but on playback the tape appeared to carry many voices. Every recording system has its own form of 'noise', and the human ear specializes in hearing human voices even when they are not there (just as the human eye is good at seeing human faces in completely non-human objects). Still, if an expert hearer can recognize some of the voices, and regards at least one of them as a genuine speaker from a past time, Raudive's electronic effect might be incorporated into an element of a machine to acquire information from the unknown world. It might form part of the 'front end' of a computer with an unconscious mind (Chapter 16).

Yet another acoustic oddity, but one which has resisted several attempts to prevent it or investigate it, is the 'direct voice' sometimes heard during séances or paranormal investigations. It is a human voice, but one whose timbre, character and style of speech differ greatly from of that of any human being present. One such voice claimed to be that of the Devil. Later it changed its style and claimed to be an angel sent to send the Devil away. During World War I, when many bereaved relatives went to mediums in the hope of making contact with those who had died, many mediums seemed to speak 'ventriloquially' by such a direct voice, and claimed that this voice was that of the dead person. I suspect that much of this was clever trickery. Kipling, who lost his own son at Loos in 1915, later wrote a disturbing poem, 'En-dor' (Chapter 15), which may have been based on a real encounter with this trade.

One interesting feature of some reports is the voice often spoke a foreign language: one unknown to the medium in the case. Indeed, almost all the ex-human entities 'on the other side' should speak such a language. The phenomenon of 'xenoglossy', as it has been called, seems to be a powerful instance of the display of knowledge not possessed by the medium, and is therefore evidence for its origin outside that medium—perhaps as information from the unknown world. One such entity apparently claimed to be ancient Egyptian, and appeared able to converse in that language. The written xenoglossy I discuss in Chapter 15 adds to the authenticity of the story. This seemingly related to medieval Glastonbury, whose apparently dead monks and construction workers spoke Low Latin or Medieval English.

Electrical effects

In the 1970s, when the Toronto Society for Psychical Research devised its project to 'invent' the ghost 'Philip', it encountered the unexpected oddity that Philip could, if asked, make the lights flicker. They illuminated the room partly by a system of lamps of different colours—they had hoped to get a visible apparition and had planned to photograph it if it appeared. To make a light flicker, you might alter the voltage driving it. This sometimes happens because of an irregularity in the voltage maintained by the power company. All the electrical apparatus supplied from that source should then behave strangely. The Toronto group did not suffer in this way; its other electrical apparatus and that in the rest of the building remained steady. To make just one bulb flicker, you would either have to make the insulator around it conducting or you would have to increase the electrical resistance of the wire supplying it. Philip once extinguished a lightbulb completely for a long time. The obvious interpretation was that it had simply failed, say by a break in its filament, but it was later found to be entirely sound. The Toronto group also noticed the strange way in which one psychic character suffered repeated failures of his rented television set. The company owning the set examined it on several occasions and found that the same small resistor had burned out. Maybe it held off a high voltage, and its resistance had briefly fallen.

This ability to alter electrical properties agrees with several related paranormal phenomena—in particular the annoying tendency of poltergeists to interfere with tape recorders or similar machinery intended to record their activities. It also agrees with the unusual abilities of a German poltergeist (in Rosenheim, Bavaria). In 1967, the local lawyer Sigmund Adam had his operations greatly degraded by dramatic changes in the electrical system. The main power supply, which was later monitored by specially installed meters, often showed wild variations, and the lighting of the office frequently failed or exploded. The telephone bill was vastly increased by calls that nobody made. When an employee was given leave, the disturbances ceased, suggesting that she was the 'focus' for the poltergeist (later she found employment elsewhere; there were strange electrical disturbances at her new office, but they died away in time).

Chemical effects

My musings here are even more speculative. I include them because we all rely on the stable properties of materials, even over long periods of time (thus stonemasons often say, 'If it will stand for ten seconds, it will stand for a thousand years'). Our whole technology assumes that properties which are essentially chemical and due to the forces between atoms (such as the strength of structural materials) never change.

So I am very interested in seeming atomic changes. Dr Bernard Grad of Mcgill University, in Montreal, once experimented with Mr Oskar Estebany, a 'healer' who discovered his unusual power while working with military animals in Hungary. Dr Grad found that wounded mice seem to heal faster if their cages had been briefly held by Mr Estebany. I cannot discover how close to the cage Mr Estebany had to come, and how long he had to remain there, to have any detectable effect. Control cages containing other wounded mice were held by other people, but interesting details of space and time again seem not to have been recorded. In another sort of test, Grad found that plant seeds grew more vigorously if Mr Estebany had held the tubes of water-based liquid they were given. A similar claim has been published by Yan Xin, also a 'healer', this time a Chinese master of the traditional 'qigong' method of medicine.

One report has it that Yan Xin may have changed the Raman spectra of the solutions. This claim astonishes me, and deserves detailed investigation. If true, it suggests to me as a chemist that the adept has altered the character not of the biological molecules dissolved in the water, but of the water itself. The Raman spectrum of water and its related infrared spectrum are both very well known. They tell chemists a lot about the forces between the atoms in its molecule, and those between the molecules themselves. Water is one of most studied of materials: it is a standard substance in numerous ways, and the stability of its various properties is universally taken for granted. Thus its freezing point and its boiling point are part of the International Temperature Scale. Its heat capacity is enshrined in the 'calorie' (the amount of heat needed to raise 1 gram of water 1 degree Celsius). Its density and the way it changes with temperature and its infrared, Raman, microwave and NMR spectra are all very well known. Innumerable compounds with accurately measured properties have known amounts of 'water of crystallization' in them. So if a healer could alter the properties of water, he or she might have a powerful effect. Most living things are largely water (the sceptical atheist J. B. S. Haldane once remarked, 'Even the Pope is 70 percent water') and most of the micro-organisms that cause disease also live in it.

So the notion that an adept might be able to alter the chemical properties of water opens a huge area of speculation. I recall a correspondence I once had with a homoeopathist. He was dismayed to find that it often seemed to work, did not understand why, and wondered whether I could suggest a reason. I failed: his account of his procedure did not suggest any sort of subtle chemistry that might have been at work. But I now wonder whether he might have been affecting the properties of his water, paranormally and unwittingly. A paper that seemed to support homoeopathy was once submitted to the scientific magazine *Nature* by the eminent biochemist Jacques Benveniste. It put John Maddox, the editor of *Nature*, in a difficult position. He did not want merely to reject the paper, as he could easily have done. Instead, in a unique editorial reaction, he employed conjurors to look for trickery in Benveniste's laboratory. The paper ultimately appeared in *Nature*[10] in 1988; Maddox defended his reaction in a number of sceptical comments that he put into that issue. Even Benveniste himself did not claim to understand his results. He merely guessed that the water might in some way have 'remembered' the molecules that were once dissolved in it. I now reckon that a brief change in the physical properties of Benveniste's water could have occurred, and this could have been revealed by the infrared or Raman spectrum of the solvent. This suggestion maintains high scientific standards: it avoids the dishonesty implied by those conjurors. Furthermore, spectroscopy is quick and simple compared with relatively complicated and unconvincing assessments of the rates of biological healing. I feel that any future biologists in the same predicament should try it.

Benveniste himself, in his musings about 'molecular memory', implies that molecules may somehow be able to hold information. This is not obviously contrary to quantum mechanics. Quantum theory may govern fundamental particles, but the accepted kinetic theory of molecular motion still allows a molecule to possess any velocity in any direction. Accordingly, it is not absurd to imagine that a molecule may also hold some element of an unlimited amount of information. It should not be restricted to a few specific quantized units of data. Like Benveniste, I cannot imagine how this might work. Current theory asserts that a molecule holds no information, and moves and spins entirely at random as a result of collisions with other molecules. The average intensity of these impacts depends on the temperature of the sample. I am free to speculate that if a molecule holds information, it does so by some sort of linkage to information in the unknown world. This notion makes sense of Benveniste's findings, and indeed of many other homoeopathic claims. It also explains the strange way in which psychometrists can sometimes acquire information from material objects (below). In Chapter 16 I glance again at the notion that molecules may somehow be able to hold information from the unknown world.

Another interesting effect, which also seems to be associated with brief changes of the forces between atoms, is the alteration of material shape. Many metals are rigid enough to be technically useful. The force required to bend a metal, the energy it stores in the process, and the force needed to leave the metal with a specific deformation after that force has been removed are important technical matters. They have been the subject of much research, and generations of engineers have come to take such findings for granted. Accordingly, the claim by a few psychics to bend metal easily, presumably by some brief and softening change in the forces between their atoms, is hard to accept. Yet there have been several psychic metal-benders (including Matthew Manning, mentioned in Chapter 9, as well as the 'spoon-bender' Uri Geller). While many frauds have been detected, I am reluctant to denounce the whole idea as clever trickery. Indeed, I suspect that the unknown world outside our diving bell can occasionally alter the forces between atoms, and thus bring about the strange effects that I have been talking about. Such effects happen, if at all, very rarely. We continue to use metals for their reliable strength, and the designers of forges and presses for metals seem not to fear for their jobs. Several other materials which we commonly regard as rigid may also be vulnerable to psychic bending. One example is the wood of the tables used by the Toronto group in 1972 (above). The paranormal 'raps' of that table sounded very different from any raps the group could make, and imply atomic changes in the wood. They used several tables in the course of their investigation, and each table was able to make these seemingly uncaused raps. They once noted that their tabletop appeared to deform, with lumps appearing in its surface 'like oranges'. This is of course impossible for wood, which in normal circumstances would break long before it could soften and deform in that way. I discuss in Chapter 9 the strange report of the Toronto workers that their wooden table could move. Influenced by the fictitious Philip, it became not only flexible, but energetically active. The Toronto table, on occasions and even in bright light, could walk, dance, and even climb. This again argues that some chemical change was going on in the leg joints of a wooden table. Again, the Toronto workers usually taped a microphone to the underside of their table to record its raps. Sometimes, often when their fictitious ghost Philip did not like a question, it fell off. Again, candies were sometimes placed on the table. They generally slid off when it was tilted even slightly, but one 'given' to Philip stayed on even at 45 degrees. This suggests to me that the adhesive chemical properties of the wooden surface could also be briefly and locally changed.

A quite different sort of chemical effect is 'thoughtography'. This is a surprising outcome of photography in which the final visible image differs from the scene the photographer thought was being recorded. In some way the unknown world has influenced or taken over the process of imaging or development. The resulting 'thoughtograph' seems to come at least partly from the mind of a person nearby.

Thoughtography appeared almost as soon as photography was invented. An image of a group of people sometimes included a figure not present on the screen or the view finder of the camera. The complicated process of development in a dark room gave many opportunities for trickery, of course. One of the most perplexing and dramatic examples of spirit photography was the achievement of the Japanese academic Tomokichi Fukurai, who in 1931 made a stack of three photographic plates, upon the centre one of which the character he employed as a medium laid a mental image. When all three plates were developed, the centre one showed that image, while the others remained blank. Clearly, the effect could not have been radiative, or all three plates would have developed in the same way.

The most interesting recent 'thoughtographer' was Ted Serios in the 1960s. His career seems to have started in a hypnotic trance, when he went on an out-of-body experience (I mention such experiences in Chapter 10). He went on several such excursions, and in one he thought to take a camera with him to make a record of the places he visited. He soon found unidentified scenes on the film. He turned his skills to photography and used the recently invented Polaroid camera—an instrument well known to many experts, and very hard to subvert. He produced, not only with his own Polaroid camera, but with ones supplied by witnesses, a long series of pictures that bore no relation to whatever was in front of the camera. They seemed instead to correspond to a thought given to him by somebody: often a 'target' image he was shown, or something he had to imagine, such as the Arc de Triomphe in Paris. In this case, the picture he produced was that of a Triumph motorcar, in which he was more interested. He also produced lots of 'blackies' (prints from which light seemed have been excluded) and 'whities' (prints seeming grossly overexposed). He often let other people operate the camera, and he made almost no attempt to prevent witnesses watching whatever he did. The only constant factor seemed to be his presence. He clearly showed some unique but unknown ability in his field. It interests me that his ability, whatever it was, seemed not only local but limited to one specific camera. Those around him were able to take entirely normal photographs, even with essentially identical Polaroid cameras. His strange ability did not spread from its target.

Ted Serios gave up his dramatic career in the early 1970s. For almost all of the rest of us, the camera seems to have been an entirely reliable object. Whenever strange images have been encountered by professional film companies, they have always judged them to come from 'double exposure'. Some people have been troubled by the unwanted (and mercifully, temporary) ability to fog any film they came near. I mention this effect in Chapters 6 and 9. It seems to have been an intriguing local effect; I know of no experiments to discover how far away it could reach, or whether any sort of screen prevented it. Sometimes an extra subject has inexplicably appeared in what was intended to be an ordinary snapshot; the widespread replacement of film by digital photodiode systems seems not so far to have created equivalent reported mysteries. I like the idea that a modern thoughtographer might come up with a whole moving image showing some scene from the unconscious mind, perhaps relayed from the unknown world, but so far we only have those enigmatic single pictures. My interpretation of the effect is that some action of the unknown world seems able to take an image in the unconscious mind of some rare adept, and transfer it somehow to the emulsion of physical film.

Materialization

One way in which the unknown world might interact with the physical one would be to create a physical object and leave it behind. What sort of things might one expect? Miraculous material objects (such as loaves and fishes) immediately suggest themselves. 'Ectoplasm', a sort of paste sometimes displayed in Victorian séances and often claimed to be remarkably strong when strength was needed, has been regarded as a non-physical material, but I have my doubts. I like the idea that the unknown world contains not only mental mysterious entities but also non-physical objects which might be made material, but I have no evidence to support this notion.

As on many previous occasions, I have allowed myself to be inspired by fiction. In 1968 Arthur C. Clarke published his novel *2001: A Space Odyssey*.[8] It featured an object found on the Moon, the so-called 'Tycho Magnetic Anomaly'. In the story it had been put there by aliens. It had properties far beyond anything possible for human technology. Thus it was so totally black that no light could ever be reflected from it, and its shape had an awesome geometrical precision. Clarke said nothing about its weight.

Other fictional stories I have read told of people who have found or have been given 'fairy gold'. This deceptive material often 'turned to withered leaves in the morning'. All this stimulates my interest in the sorts of stuff that we might expect to find created in the unknown world and materialized in the physical one.

A material object which has merely been moved around (an apport in the jargon) might not be affected by the experience. Poltergeists sometimes seem to have a liking for moving particular objects: bottles or stones, for example. Sometimes they seem to release lots of water. This might just be a cooling effect (I discuss in Chapter 10 how haunting seems to lower the temperature); water can be extracted from the air by cooling it below the dew point. On some occasions, enough water has been released for analysis, which has indicated a local source. This of course suggests that the poltergeist had just been moving existing water around.

Objects which seem to have been moved through a solid surface (teleports in the jargon) suggest further tests. Thus I have read of an egg which was moved from a closed container to a volume outside it, and of a snowball which a Polish medium claimed to have teleported into a closed room on a cold winter's day! Such an event, if genuine, suggests a sudden change in the physical properties of some region of the room or container, so the object was able to go through it. These surfaces might give useful clues as to what had happened. The most significant event would be a true materialization: the sudden appearance of a physical object. Several were recorded in Victorian séances, but I am inclined to dismiss them as trickery. One medium got rid of alleged materializations by eating them—which I regard as a neat way of disposing of a fraud.

There is one obvious outcome of materialization, which I have never heard of. If a material object were suddenly made to appear in our world by some paranormal effect, it would produce a loud 'bang!' as the air was expelled from the volume it occupied. Similarly, if a material object were made to disappear paranormally, there would be another sudden 'bang!' as the air rushed in to occupy the volume it had vacated. Various religious miracles have been claimed to have created or destroyed material objects, but no accompanying noises have even been reported. A quiet materialization implies a slow one, so that the displaced air is gradually moved away without obvious noise. Again, I have never read any reports of such gradual miracles.

Another interesting possible connection between the physical world and the non-physical one is the way that certain 'sensitives' claim to be able to handle an object and deduce things about its previous owner. An object that the previous owner regarded as a 'possession', say a watch, a pen, a cufflink or a ring, often seems very informative. This ability is sometimes known as 'psychometry'. Since it deals with the way a sensitive may acquire information about an object, and does not imply any insight or change in its chemical nature, it may be a branch of clairvoyance and nothing to do with chemistry. I mention it in this chemical section essentially for convenience. Animals, of course, pick up information about objects all the time using their acute sense of smell. Humans may do it too (the physicist Richard Feynman claimed to be able to tell from its smell if a book had recently been handled), but they may also be able to pick up some sort of information from the object about its history. I am reminded of the claim I made in Chapter 7 that some objects might, if thermally isolated, cool a bit faster towards the low temperature of the unknown world. The author Browning has recorded that a psychometrist to whom he had given a cufflink to hold was inspired to exclaim 'Murder!' The cufflink came from a great-uncle of Browning's who had indeed been violently killed.

Again, dowsing has occasionally recorded great triumphs, but has also failed critical tests. As with many 'psychic' abilities, skill in it is distributed unevenly and it is hard to learn. Dowsers often hold rods of some sort and generally claim to be aware of them twitching or moving when they get above something interesting. I suspect that in fact it is the unconscious mind of the dowser that becomes aware of the interesting information, and acts on his or her hands to make the rods move. The whole effect seems to be driven by the unconscious mind of the dowser, which drives his or her hands in response. The action strongly resembles the way in which information can be gathered by planchette or by automatic writing (Chapter 16). With the conscious mind distracted, the unconscious one can dominate the movements of hand

and arm. I have read the claim that a master dowser, directly aware of information entering his unconscious mind anyway, does not need rods. He or she may be alerted to the local geochemistry of the site by information held about it in the unknown world. That information might even include its geohistory. Thus Jeffrey Goodman has claimed that a sensitive from Oregon helped him to locate a site near Flagstaff, Arizona, which contained a large number of objects dating back to a human settlement of 25,000 BC or before. I have also heard of a dowser who acquired information about an object thousands of miles away.

Many 'possessions' studied by psychometrists are very intimate—rings, cufflinks, etc. Other objects (for example, tools which are just as firmly possessed by one individual and are only used by him or her) may not be so intimate. It occurs to me that false teeth, or metal tooth fillings, or even grave bones, are also highly intimate objects which might somehow acquire information about their owner. I have never heard of any 'sensitive' reacting to such objects, but they are widely available. They might be worth a study.

If an alleged non-physical or psychometrically significant object came my way, I would record its size, weight and nature very precisely and study it for a long time to be aware of any slow changes. I might then put it under high vacuum, heat part of it radiatively and apply a strong electric field. Any physical object would emit electrons, and I would be interested to discover if they had the same charge and mass as the electrons we know about. I also like the idea of cleaning the object, to remove anything from its surface (such as possible smell-substances). With a coherent solid object, such as a ring, it might even be possible to remove the top thousand or so atoms using a dilute acid. It would be interesting to discover if the resulting denuded object still stirred notions in the mind of a psychometrist. The molecules of the object might, of course, be somehow connected to information in the unknown world (above), but I cannot suggest a way of studying this possibility. It interests me that many reported paranormal effects include or consist of, brief changes in the forces between atoms which we which we usually take as reliably constant. For example, pychokinesis and poltergeists (the mechanical laws), levitation (the law of gravity), walking tables and spoon-bending (strength of materials), and thoughtography (chemical effects on a photographic plate).

12

Unscientific but Widespread Human Beliefs

At this point in my text, I am aware of having to make an abrupt change of mental gear. Previously, my approach has been essentially intellectual. In considering some paranormal claim, I have asked myself, Is this likely to be true? Should I take it seriously? If so, I try to see if an extension of existing physical theory could accommodate it. Now I have to approach notions that have a strong human or emotional element, while retaining as much as I can of that detached and scientific stance. This often seems very difficult. Many of those who oppose the theory of evolution, for example, do so essentially because it offends their religious feelings. They do not care about its likelihood, but find it emotionally repellant. So it is with some diffidence that I begin to compare my notions of the unknown world with the informal beliefs that many people seem to hold about themselves.

The two show some interesting parallels. In proposing an 'unknown world outside our diving bell', I may also

Why Are We Conscious? A Scientist's Take on Consciousness and Extrasensory Perception
David E. H. Jones

ISBN 978-981-4774-32-1 (Hardcover), 978-1-315-16688-9 (eBook)
www.panstanford.com

be supporting the existence of a theological world. It is a common religious dogma that God is everywhere (omnipresent). Accordingly, many religious believers feel that they can pray to God anywhere and can also conduct anywhere acts of worship for Him to be aware of. That theological world may also contain paradise and hell, which many people reckon are occupied by the souls of human beings after their bodily death. I must acknowledge the possibility that this theological world is some sort of human interpretation of my unknown world.

Thus, among the inhabitants of the unknown world outside our diving bell, there may be entities remarkably similar to ones which many people already half-believe in informally: angels, devils, the souls of dead people, and so on. Two of the cases which I later describe in more detail (Chapter 15) seem to assume the existence of a theological world beyond the physical space we know about. One of them is the recovery by Bond and Alleyne of useful information about the long-destroyed Edgar Chapel at Glastonbury, apparently from the souls of dead monks who knew the building in its days of glory. The other is the attempt, seemingly by the dead men Frederick Myers, Edmund Gurney and Henry Sidgwick, to transfer information about that after-death world and their current state in it to the physical world. Their efforts exploited clever 'cross-correspondences' transferred to selected mediums. The fictitious ghost 'Philip' (Chapters 6 and 11), created in 1972 by members of the Toronto Society for Psychical Research, may have been a counter-example. Eight persons, none of them claiming any psychic ability, created Philip and were able to get table rappings and table movements from him (though not the visible apparition they had been hoping for). Philip was completely synthetic, and no 'spiritual' entity seems to have been behind him. My sense is that the Toronto group had made some sort of contact with the unknown world, but not with any human after-death entities in it—if such there be.

Accordingly the unknown non-material world 'outside our diving bell', though it is currently undetectable by instrumental means, may contain many things that many people would like to believe in. Even theologians admit that nobody has yet devised a religious creed that both makes sense and fits the facts as we know them. I am reminded of the Australian aboriginal suspicions of what Christian missionaries declared: 'The god-men say when die go sky / Through pearly gates where river flow, / The god-men say when die we fly / Just like eagle, hawk and crow. / Might be, might be— / But I don't know.' Yet those missionaries were very firm in what they believed and what they were trying to teach. That firmness is still extremely strong. Religious terrorism is distressingly common these days. Adherents of one religion often kill those of another. By contrast, almost nobody would spill half a pint of blood for any claim from physical science or paranormal study.

I here acknowledge a possible theological interpretation of the unknown world, but do not assume, endorse or deduce anything from it. I try to stay with Valérian 'public truths', for example those of paranormalism and psychiatry. Paranormalism is in essence a large number of anecdotes supported by a web of laboratory experiments. It often depends on some unusual person, such as a 'star guesser' with the rare ability to guess better than chance. Psychiatry is not a science at all but a technology: it exists to counter various forms of mental illness. And yet one of its hypotheses, that of the unconscious mind, seems to me among the great guesses of the 1900s. It has been applied to the higher animals, and plays a crucial part in my guesses about consciousness.

Even so, it is with some reluctance and uncertainty that I start to compare my notions of the unknown world with relatively informal and highly unscientific social beliefs. I am somewhat encouraged by a remark due to Gilbert K. Chesterton: 'The real trouble with this world of ours is not that it is an unreasonable one. The trouble is that it is nearly reasonable, but not quite.' A few of those unreasonable notions have been greatly changed by physical science. Thus a few centuries ago many people used to imagine, for example, that the universe had been specially created for humanity. The earth was taken as flat, maybe cake-shaped. God made it for men to live on. Above it was the sky, which shaded into heaven where He and the angels lived, and to which your soul went after death if you had been good enough. It was possible to make occasional contact with God through prayer, revelation and the holy books. These reinforced His notions of virtue and sin (He had pretty much invented both and preferred the former to the latter) and His purposes for humankind. Below the surface of the earth was hell, where it was hot and very nasty, where the devil ruled, and where your soul went after death if you had not been good enough. All this made both moral and physical sense. We would all like to believe that we have souls, that human life has some moral purpose, and that the world was created as our home.

Imperfect and essentially prescientific knowledge seemed to support such views. Below ground it is indeed hot (volcanoes and so on reinforced that belief), and nobody had gone far into the sky to have data on heaven. Both the ascension to heaven and the descent to hell seemed to suggest that Up was good and Down was bad. As Kipling wrote, 'Down to Gehenna or up to the Throne, / He travels fastest who travels alone'. There was also a common notion that everything was very short-lived. Many people believed that God had made the whole thing about 6000 years ago and that some great change (such as the second coming of Christ) would happen very soon.

With the rise of physical science, all such traditional beliefs have been questioned, and many have been abandoned. Thus geology has disposed of hell—the earth is indeed hot inside, but it is solid—and astronomy has found no trace of heaven. When the Russians put the first man into orbit, they claimed that he did not see God up there. (That man was Yuri Gagarin, and C. S. Lewis responded to his remark by saying that it would be like Hamlet going into the attic of his castle looking for Shakespeare. Verbal transcripts dispute Gagarin's alleged statement.) The Russian space agency seems to have been attacking a notion of heaven in which a few people still believed. Most no longer saw it as a physical place in the sky. This abandoned belief may not merely reflect that cynical claim for Christianity: 'Pie in the sky when you die'. It may have been reinforced by the epic *Paradise Lost*, in which John Milton imagined Vulcan being thrown out of heaven by Jove. His fall to Earth took a whole day: 'From morn to noon he fell, from noon to dewy eve, / A summer's day, and with the setting sun / Dropt from the zenith.' French[13] has calculated the height of heaven from this passage. He takes the day as being 17.5 hours, the longest day of the English summer, and allows for the weakening of gravity with height. He gets about 10^5 km. Astronomy and space exploration have not, of course, found anything at or near this height.

A further change is our sense of time. Most of us now accept the cosmological notion that that the universe has existed for billions of years. Similarly, our sense of the future also now extends into a distant remoteness. As the *Cambridge Encyclopaedia* says about the world of astronomy, 'It will all be over in fifty billion years.' Nonetheless, one major puzzle haunts every single human being. Science has nothing to say about it, and religious dogmas have filled the void unconvincingly. My notions of the unknown world and the nature of consciousness also seem relevant to the question. It has always been very important to humanity. What happens when we die?

In writing this book, I have always felt a connection between the unknown world outside our diving bell and the limits to human life. We all fear death, but try not to think of it. 'Old Man River', written by Oscar Hammerstein II for the American musical *Show Boat*, is sung by a man who sometimes feels 'tired of living and scared of dying'. In his popular poem on the death of his cat, Henry Forbes ('Hal') Summers, wrote, 'Well died, my old cat', thus raising the fear of death in every reader. One reaction to that fear is religious. As Arthur Clough wrote in 1850, 'And almost every one when age, / Disease or sorrows strike him, / Inclines to think there is a God, / Or something very like Him.' That Victorian eccentric Edward Lear once wrote a poem about himself. It goes in part 'He reads but he cannot speak Spanish, / he cannot abide ginger-beer. / Ere the days of his pilgrimage vanish, / How pleasant to know Mr Lear!' Sadly, the days of all our pilgrimages must vanish.

Anyway, my argument here is that death need not be a total end. Some sort of information in the unconscious mind, held in the unknown world, may survive it. Myers's brave book, *Human Personality and Its Survival of Bodily Death*, came out in 1903, two years after his own death in 1901. He seems after death, and with the dead spirits of two other members of the Society, Gurney and Sidgwick, to have set up subtle 'cross-correspondences' from beyond the grave to selected mediums (Chapter 15). These have resisted full interpretation, but seem to imply that for some people at least, a useful amount of intellectual power may survive physical death. A great deal of information, held by people who have lived, also seems to survive as well.

The thesis of this book is that information exists in the unknown world, but I do not know what form it might take. I suspect that human beings have access to more information than we can hold in the human brain (Appendix D), and that some of it exists in non-material form in the unknown world outside our diving bell. My feeling is that while we are alive, we have some sort of special access to that information. After our death, some of it may continue to exist in the unknown world. It may be associated with, or be held by, some entity in that world which can transfer some of it to another unconscious mind. Telepathy (which I discuss in Chapter 8) may be a form of such transfer in which both unconscious minds are alive.

Any information-holding entity is, I feel, free to wander in that unknown world, at the sort of velocities I muse about in Chapter 7. While the human being who 'owns' the information is alive, however, it has to stay in contact with him or her. I am reminded of one old definition of staying alive: 'keeping body and soul together'. This supports my expectation that, while a human being is alive, any information held in the unconscious mind in non-material form is always close to the living body in physical space. Indeed, in theological terms it may be held by a personal 'guardian angel'—an entity whose nature I cannot guess, but perhaps exists, and if so, probably deserves that name. In this text I merely feel that if we hold at least some information not in the brain but in non-material form in the unknown world, then it has to stay near its owner and must follow that owner around somehow.

The fate of human consciousness after death

In this section of text, I look briefly at some 'theological' claims about the unknown world as a possible container of elements of humanity after death. Such claims are not implied in my musings, but they are widely asserted. In many traditional beliefs, death is not the end of everything. A dead person releases a 'soul' which retains much of the identity of the dier. The soul might go 'Up' to heaven or 'Down' to hell. Its direction seems a moral matter. Some versions of Christianity have a recording angel compiling a record of every human life, to be scanned when the time comes for judgement. This would be a vast task. Even in the Middle Ages when the recording angel was first proposed, there were about a billion human beings living. The angel had to accumulate the life history of each of them in sufficient detail to submit the record to God for judgement. I feel that even angelic power would struggle with such a task. If I were a theologian, I might suggest that each personal 'guardian angel' should have the job of making the record for that person. Heinrich Heine saw the whole matter as very simple. Everyone, he felt, will go to heaven. His famous last words were 'God will forgive me; it's His job'. Yet divine judgement may be more subtle than this. It seems to be a sort of end-of-term exam. Different versions of theology give different weightings to your past beliefs and your past actions. It is not clear if faith trumps work, or vice versa. The pass mark of the examination is even more unclear. If it is 99 percent, only almost perfect saints will go to heaven. One advantage of being a martyr for your faith is that if you are killed in a sufficiently painful or dramatic manner, God may overlook the sins of your previous life and push your score above the pass mark, so that you go to heaven. Islamic 'suicide bombers' may have this notion somewhere in their fanatical minds. On the other hand, if that pass mark is 1 percent, almost everybody will go to heaven anyway. Christian theology seems to say nothing about the average person, who might score about 50 percent in the exam. Purgatory, not as nasty as hell but not as nice as heaven, might be the right place for such folk.

Re-entering a living body: reincarnation

An alternative notion, common in religions such as Buddhism, is that a dying person may go neither to heaven nor to hell, or purgatory, but may be reborn in physical form, 'reincarnated'. He or she would have his or her consciousness transferred to a creature then being born. In all probability, this would be some animal. The transfer might be a rapid form of judgement, so that someone wicked, with a low moral mark in the exam, would be punished by being reincarnated as a lower animal. Alternatively, the transfer might depend on one's feelings at the moment of death—a worry, for many people would be extremely dismayed or frightened at that moment. If the transfer depends entirely on timing, anyone dying at a specific instant might be transferred to whatever was being born at that instant. I have failed to discover any theory about what the reincarnation system is or how it works, but to ensure that it catches every dying individual, it must be everywhere. (No astronaut has yet died on the Moon, but the reincarnation system would have to be able to accommodate the sad possibility and implement a decision.) If the system was judgemental, it might look around for a birth that fitted the dying person and the about-to-be released soul. It might plan to let the reincarnated soul continue whatever work it had in progress, or it might want to release it from the whole business of reincarnation, and let it enter 'nirvana' (a Buddhist version of heaven).

Suppose the released soul were transferred to an animal. Would that animal be aware of its lowness, know that certain other animals are superior, and understand that it should begin the long climb back up to virtue? Or might it think, as Robert Frost once wrote of a wasp, 'Poor egotist, he has no way of knowing / But he's as good as anybody going!' And imagine that the new animal has to live in a tribe of other animals without an inbuilt moral purpose. If it were a rat (say), it might ignore the promptings of virtue. It might just get on with ratty life in accordance with its instincts.

If the released human soul were transferred to another human baby, further problems could arise. Such human-to-human reincarnation is widely accepted in many communities. Sometimes a pregnant woman has an 'announcing dream' in which the previous identity of her forthcoming child is given or implied (I discuss dreams in Chapter 10.) That reincarnation is often reinforced when a new child begins to speak, maybe at the age of two or three, and recalls the previous life it lived. The new child generally forgets that previous life, or stops speaking about it, around the ages of five to eight. Sometimes its memories and claims of its preceding life can be verified, and turn out to apply to a person known to have previously died. One complication is that the previous death may not have happened at the moment the new child was born or conceived. It may be that a soul has to wait in some sort of 'limbo' until a suitable birth occurs, or can be set up. In communities which accept human reincarnation as common, a delay between about six months and four years seems acceptable. Where and what is that reincarnation limbo, and what other inhabitants might it have? My simplest guess is that a soul awaiting reincarnation does not go into any sort of limbo at all, but just occupies the same space as any other soul. Nonetheless, that delay intrigues me. Thus in Buddhist tradition the noted Tibetan Lama Gedun Drub died in 1474, but his reincarnated successor did not appear till a child named

Sangye Chophel was born in 1476. Drub's soul must have been stored somewhere for about two years. The notion of reincarnation, of course, reduces the huge number of human souls (10^{11}), which I calculate in Chapter 10. The facts of human birth and death also fit the idea that a smaller set of souls just goes round and round in an endless cycle of reincarnations ('bound on the wheel', as the Lama said in Kipling's *Kim*). This notion may reduce our fear of death, but increase our concern for the future of humanity. We have, of course, absolutely no knowledge of when or into what sort of body a person might be reborn (the great physicist Enrico Fermi pondered that he might 'come back as an elephant'). Some interpretations of Buddhism dislike reincarnation. Thus the Puri sect in eastern India has a huge vehicle (known to Europeans as a 'juggernaut') carrying their idol Jagnannath. Fanatics of the sect throw themselves under the vehicle to be crushed to death. They hope that this means of demise will release them from the cycle of reincarnation.

Reincarnation implies the existence of a human soul which carries not only a unique 'identity' and a continuation of consciousness, but a great deal of information—memories of the world it recently inhabited. It must also carry, or at least have access to, the memories it amassed in all previous lives. The notion of repeated reincarnation seems to imply access to an ever-growing number of memories of previous lives. Even if some of them were the memories of a rat, they still add to some expanding amount of information. Where does it all go? I dislike the idea that the soul can get full of memory and has to throw data away. I prefer the assumption that it has an effectively bottomless permanent receptacle for memory in its non-physical abode. This corresponds to the idea that the unknown world can hold a large but quite undefined amount of information, and the unconscious mind of a sensitive may be able to access some of it. This fits the story I report in Chapter 11, in which a sensitive in Oregon helped an archaeological team in its search for an old site.

Psychiatric patients have sometimes reported 'memories' of being in the womb, and even of being born. This sort of claim has been advocated as an explanation of 'enlightenment' (Chapter 15). It is opposed by the medical argument that the brain and the memory nerves are not fully formed and functional at the time we are born. They only start to work properly at the age of about three—which is why our earliest conscious memory is typically of some event around that time. Such claims make more sense if the memory of being born is stored not in the brain at all, but in the unknown world. It is accessed by the brain later through the unconscious mind, which of course distorts it.

Another aspect of reincarnation, though commonly looked for, seems contradicted by current genetic knowledge. This is the idea that a person may be born with some sort of defect or birthmark also present in his or her previous incarnation. It is worth trying to discover whether the new individual has such a distinguishing mark. This suggestion has to be nonsense. There is no way that such a defect or birthmark could get into the DNA of the new baby. The DNA of any baby is simply a subset of that of its parents. However, heredity is never perfect. Many slightly defective people, or ones with birthmarks, merely represent a slight irregularity in the way that their DNA was copied from that of their parents. During a woman's pregnancy, many 'quality control' checks are carried out automatically by her biology (so a woman who suffers a miscarriage may in fact be rejecting a substandard baby).

I know of only one Western claim of reincarnation. It was made on behalf of an American woman, Virginia

Tighe. It was published in 1952 by Morey Bernstein in a book titled *The Search for Bridey Murphy*. Morey Bernstein was an amateur hypnotist. His book claimed that Mrs Tighe, born in 1923, was the reincarnation of Bridey Murphy, an Irish woman of the 1800s who died in 1864. On my thesis here, she would have spent some 59 years in limbo but would have no conscious memory of it. Even so, my sense is that if human reincarnation were at all common, it would be much more widely reported and accepted, and clues to it would exist in many people's memories. I recall Bob Dylan's song about the wretched Hollis Brown, a failing American farmer who spent his last lone dollar on seven shotgun shells. The result was 'seven people dead On a South Dakota farm / Somewhere in the distance / There's seven new people born'.

13

Organizations and Unusual People

The decline of magic

IN PRIMITIVE SOCIETIES, ALMOST EVERYBODY believed in magic. This is not inherently absurd. Indeed, the science fiction writer Robert Heinlein has defined magic as technology which you do not understand. If (like some primitive people) you understand almost nothing, then almost everything is magic. The recent rise of science has had several beneficial effects. First, of course, it has granted us an enormous increase in our standard of living (I am now thinking not only of such blessings as electricity, artificial light, clean water and cheap energy, but of biochemical wonders like anaesthetics and contraceptives). Second, it has made a lot of the physical world understandable. Third, its sheer power has shown us the benefits of accurate and careful observation and experiment, and the steady technical development this makes possible. One important consequence of this scientific rise has been the

Why Are We Conscious? A Scientist's Take on Consciousness and Extrasensory Perception
David E. H. Jones

ISBN 978-981-4774-32-1 (Hardcover), 978-1-315-16688-9 (eBook)
www.panstanford.com

almost total demolition of magic. Almost nobody now believes in it seriously; almost everybody reckons that a demonstration of magic is fraudulent trickery; almost all religions are now apologetic about the alleged 'miracles' described in their writings. Those scientific 'recipes which always work' seem to have conquered everything.

Yet magic is still socially very popular. Many people would like to believe in it: hence (perhaps) the great success of the Harry Potter books. These have been denounced in some African and Arab countries, and even in some American states, for 'encouraging belief in witchcraft'. I suspect that a tiny residue of genuine magic still exists in reality. Some people consistently demonstrate strange abilities denied to the rest of us, and not all of them are clever tricksters. Out on the rims of the multiple Gaussian 'bell-shaped curves' of human nature (Appendix A), we find a few people with highly unusual abilities. Here are the 'star guessers' of the paranormal laboratory who can occasionally guess better than chance. Here are the psychic mediums who can sometimes levitate things, the psychokineticists who can sometimes make things move without touching them, the thoughtographers who can sometimes put a mental image on a photographic plate: all those for whom, as Hamlet said, 'there are more things in Heaven and Earth, Horatio, / Than are dreamt of in your philosophy'. Many of these achievements may just be clever tricks, but a few may reveal glimpses of the world outside our diving bell. Normal people often just dismiss the whole topic as so much 'anecdotal evidence', probably fraudulent and in any case utterly demolished by modern science. Indeed, the whole business of magic is dense with fraud and clever conjuring. Those who are sceptical of the entire field do not have to face any powerful evidence against them. Yet I feel that people with strange abilities may at least dent the diving bell that encloses most of us. Accordingly, a book such as this one, which guesses at the existence of a world outside our known physical universe, does not automatically denounce the claims of magic.

'Magical' organizations: churches

The greatest and most dreadful aspect of human fate is the inevitability of personal death. To intercede on behalf of the dead, and to help the living, almost every society invented Gods. Social 'churches' sprang up to influence those aspects of human life that were felt to be 'in the lap of the Gods'. The civil power had to maintain a delicate stance towards such organizations. Edward Gibbon wrote that in Roman society, all religions 'were considered by the people as equally true; by the philosopher as equally false; and by the magistrate as equally useful'. Nonetheless, formal churches (often claiming to have been established by the human figurehead who started the religion of that church) came to have strong social power. They often constructed imposing buildings such as cathedrals, temples, synagogues and mosques. Their function seems at least partly social; they provide a setting in which believers can congregate together. (This is not surprising: we are social beings.) Each religious organization has officials, such as priests, bishops and imams.

Europe was much influenced by Christianity. In the Middle Ages, the Roman Catholic Church developed a lot of civil power. It claimed to have been founded by Peter, a disciple of Jesus of Nazareth. Its head, the Pope, had as much authority as many a European monarch. Later the Protestant reformation founded many rival Christian churches, and the idea developed that the connection between man and God was a one-to-one relationship. The Christian Bible, which for the benefit of the Roman

Catholic Church had been translated from Greek into Latin (the Vulgate), was further translated into many vernacular tongues for the benefit of ordinary people. (One reason for keeping it in a socially unintelligible language was that if common people could read it, they would discover that unofficial notions such as indulgences and purgatory were not in it.) Despite the notion that man should deal directly with God, the protestant churches continued to be social organizations. They continued to have buildings, appoint officials and develop congregations. The slogan 'Cut out the middleman! Deal direct with the Maker!' may have inspired enthusiasts for private worship, but did not disband the churches.

Religious beliefs were often codified into a 'creed', frequently expressed in a fairly coherent text. Usually each church, despite its tendency to split into theological divisions, had a common core of belief. Thus the Christian one has God at the top, with His angels below, and below that a range of good souls, all in heaven. In the middle is human society, whose people may aspire to go up, but fear to go down. For below there is hell, governed by the devil who commands its content of the souls of sinners. The whole thing lasts for ever. No artist has made either heaven or hell seem convincing, though the latter has been depicted with more gusto. Bertrand Russell recalled that when during World War I he went to prison, a warder asked him his religion. He replied 'agnostic'. The warder sighed, and said, 'There are many religions, but I suppose they all worship the same God.' This remark, said Russell, kept him cheerful for about a week. Here I allow an even wider spread of religious beliefs. Even so, many of the major religions seem to posit a very organized structure for the theological world. It interests me that many religious people do not bother with the lower levels of heaven. Some prayers are directed at specific saints, but many people pray directly to God at the top. It is not obvious that praying is evidence for the existence of a theological world, though many people have reported the sense that something was somehow listening to their prayer. A cynical saying is, 'If you talk to God, that's prayer. If God talks to you, that's schizophrenia.'

The conventional religions seem to assume that God knows the content of every human mind. The religions made this claim even when God was thought of as living in a relatively distant celestial heaven. Thus the Christian book of common prayer claims of God that for Him 'all hearts be open, all desires known, and from whom no secrets are hid'. There seems not to have been any theological explanation of how this information could be transmitted to God in His heaven. Indeed, if God is everywhere anyway ('omnipresent' in the theological jargon) the heavenly apparatus to study humanity seems needless. With the later invention of the human unconscious mind, information and feelings not even known to their owner are, on this interpretation, known to God.

Despite formal churches, many citizens continued to believe in informal 'magic'. The Christian Bible has an old testament which salutes the Jewish prophets, but deplores witches, wizards and those who practice occult divination or have familiar spirits. Yet in medieval times almost every village in Britain contained a witch or a wizard, to help the locals with unexpected problems. I imagine that they kept their ears open for useful social gossip and were probably a better first port of call than the local church.

In the 1600s, British law moved dramatically against witchcraft—indeed the modern word 'witch hunt', denoting an irrational drive against some socially unpopular person or cause, derives from this period. I have read of the social arrangement in which everything is illegal, but the authorities only move against actions which seem to them undesirable (this resembles the lawless societies of all social animals and some humans; Chapter 5). Even in a very legal society like that of Britain, many more crimes are committed than are ever prosecuted. 'Police discretion' decides informally which crimes leave the sort of evidence which can be presented to a court, or which are serious enough to be worth going after. The 'zero tolerance' theory of policing is an interesting alternative strategy.

Keith Thomas has argued that the 'witch hunts' of the 1600s were due to the relatively sudden competition faced by the Roman Catholic Church. This church had its own magic rituals and charms (exorcism, holy relics, the mass, talismans, etc). During the 1500s, it was strongly challenged by Protestantism, which was far less magical. Martin Luther's famous altercation with the Pope started in 1517. A few decades later King Henry VIII of Britain made the Protestant Church that of England and set in train the destruction of the Roman Catholic monasteries. In the 1640s the official British 'witchfinder' Matthew Hopkins was very active. Witchcraft, of course, had always been illegal in Britain, but until the 1600s, prosecutions resulting from claims about it were relatively rare. Once Catholic magic was no longer freely available, many people relied even more heavily on informal local magic. The authorities began to take notice, and legal accusations often resulted. Even so about 50 percent of the accused were acquitted.

The Catholic Church also faced competition on the European continent. Indeed, that witch finder's 'textbook', the 'malleus maleficarum', was a German product. It seems to have been derived from the Catholic Inquisition, implied that witchcraft was evil because of a supposed pact with the Devil, and appeared in English translation only centuries later.

The witch hunt declined dramatically in the 1700s. The British Witchcraft Act was repealed in 1736. Long before that, it had become very hard to mount a prosecution in the courts. The rise of science and rationalism may simply have made the authorities too sceptical. Other social changes probably played an important part as well. A rising standard of living reduced the sudden desperation, which often made unfortunate people run towards magic. Furthermore, the invention of probability theory and the improvements in social statistical mathematics allowed an insurance industry to develop. This offered an alternative reaction to unexpected disaster.

Unusual people

Napoleon is said once to have listed the abilities he looked for in his generals. Many such qualities relating to military competence, but he also wanted his generals 'lucky'. Luck seems not to be a consistent or reliable human quality. The gambling industry is based on the proposition that none of us is either lucky or unlucky; we are all equally governed by the laws of chance. It seems to be doing very well.

Nonetheless, Napoleon may have been onto something. We are all different, and a few of us may indeed be 'lucky'. As so often, I have allowed myself to be inspired by fiction. Larry Niven's classic science fiction story 'Ringworld' of 1970 has a heroine, Teena Brown, whose crucial characteristic is that she is 'lucky'. She has some sort of knack, so that the innumerable small chances that dominate human life tend to come out in her favour. She is a good example of the wide spread of human qualities: not just height and weight, but intellectual, emotional and personal attitudes too.

Most of us are normal members of the human race, but a few extreme people stand out as notables. They may make commanding inventors, business bosses, politicians, artists, or experimental or theoretical scientists. I feel that such unusual individuals have a rare and valuable ability well away from the centre of any human Gaussian bell (I discuss the Gaussian distribution in Appendix A). If their gift is psychic, they may become effective mediums, or commanding 'star guessers' in parapsychology.

I greatly admire such rarities. My admiration has to be balanced, of course, by great suspicion—for many of them are also clever fraudsters. Yet some seem to be genuine. They are often able to guess a bit better than chance, or guess the future more accurately than you would expect. They may claim to receive messages from another world, or be able to initiate psychokinesis. Such unusual people often seem to outflank those 'recipes which always work'. Their rare abilities may vary unpredictably, possibly depending on their mental attitude at the time, but in the right circumstances they can sometimes do things which ordinary mortals cannot do. If their gifts lean towards psychic ability, they may appear in the paranormal laboratory as 'star guessers'. Helmut Schmidt once searched for star guessers among many normal chance-bound people and reckoned that they might constitute 1 percent or less of the population at large.

The beginning of spiritualism

The spiritual studies that interest me began pretty much in the 1800s. Spiritualism as a movement seems to have started in Hydesville, USA, in 1848. A poltergeist manifested itself in the Fox household there. A family daughter, Kate Fox, seems to have felt that the poltergeist was the Devil himself (who traditionally has a cleft foot). She addressed him: 'Do as I do, Mr Splitfoot,' and clapped her hands. The poltergeist replied with rapping sounds.

Mrs Fox asked, 'Are you a spirit? If you are, rap twice.' She got two raps in reply. She started a sort of conversation based on raps. Spiritualism spread fast and is now established in many countries. It exists in effect as one of the many denominations of Christianity, although it emphasizes (what is indeed an aspect of Christian doctrine) that human beings survive death. Its special claim is that dead people are still alive in the 'spirit world' and, thanks to its expertise, can sometimes communicate with those who are alive in the physical one. Unlike many Christian denominations, it runs a newspaper (*Psychic News*) which has thousands of readers.

14

Mediumship, the Societies for Psychical Research, and Star Guessers

Mediumship

I HAVE DESCRIBED BEFORE (Chapters 6 and 11) how in 1972 the Toronto Society for Psychical Research set up a group who 'invented' the fictitious ghost Philip. The idea was that several normal people acting in concert might achieve the same sort of psychic power that one medium could command. They would, of course, have to achieve the right sort of closeness and ability to relax with each other. In the event, the group consisted of eight people, none of whom claimed any psychic ability, and none of whom acted as leader. The Society hoped to turn an unpredictable personal skill into a repeatable group technique: one of those 'recipes which always work'. So far, it seems not to have done so. No system of organizing a group into one with psychic powers has yet been published. Unusual

Why Are We Conscious? A Scientist's Take on Consciousness and Extrasensory Perception
David E. H. Jones

ISBN 978-981-4774-32-1 (Hardcover), 978-1-315-16688-9 (eBook)
www.panstanford.com

psychic ability continues to remain the rare and valuable possession of single individuals. Such people are often known as 'mediums'; the word implies a channel through which some sort of spiritual influence can easily flow. One of the people who helped to start the spiritualism movement, Kate Fox herself, later became an important medium.

A medium seems often seems able to make some sort of contact with people now dead, who are often considered to have some sort of continued existence 'on the other side'. The field is naturally dense with tricksters and frauds of all kinds. I have read that in reality true mediums are as rare as great achievers in any other field. We are lucky if half a dozen of them are born in a century.

The single 'mediums' that I discuss here are, I reckon, out on some rim of the multiple Gaussian distribution which is human nature. Mediums often become aware of their gifts through some sort of internal prompting. Indeed, many have claimed to know, and in some way to be activated through, a spiritual controller 'on the other side'. Thus the medium Gladys Osborne Leonard usually worked through a controller 'Feda', apparently a family ancestor, who claimed to have died in childbirth around 1800. The medium Maurice Barbanelle alleged that he worked through a controller called 'Silver Birch'. Leonora Piper had a recently dead controller named George Pellew.

It is not obvious to me what the function of a controller might be. The whole idea has been denounced as incoherent and irrelevant, but I can make a guess. If, as I have calculated in Chapter 10, there are about 10^{11} human souls in the spiritual world, a medium might indeed need the assistance of some sort of spirit controller to select just one of them. This guess does not seem to be supported by the statements made by mediums about their controllers. Thus mediums do not appear to be overwhelmed by an unusually large number of contacts 'on the other side'. Neither do controllers seem to work at selecting one spirit out of a huge number of possible contenders. Collectively, however, those many reported 'controllers' suggest that their world contains a lot of entities, though not perhaps 10^{11} of them. The Society for Psychical Research naturally made contact with many British Victorian mediums. After their deaths the Society members Myers, Gurney and Sidgwick appear to have sent many 'cross-correspondence' messages to them. Many of these mediums were able to take down the messages by 'automatic writing' (Chapter 15). Those messages were sent between about 1903 to 1930.Then and later, attempts were made to combine them into a coherent statement about the world the dead members were now in. However, the cross-correspondence strategy, though very clever, seems not to have succeeded. Those deceased members of the Society for Psychical Research had great trouble even in establishing their identities and were quite unable to provide a useful description of the world they inhabited. If they had any representation in the unknown world, that world was, as I have surmised about the physical world 'outside our diving bell', very weakly coupled to the physical one.

Mediums real and fraudulent often acquire a large range of 'clients', typically bereaved persons anxious to get a message from, or to send one to, a dead relative. Millions of people died in World War I, and a large trade grew up to service the hopes of surviving relatives. Many mediums thus came to have many 'clients' who came to them. The typical response of the medium was to generate some sort of message. This might be delivered verbally if the medium was conscious but aware of an incoming message, or the medium could go into some sort of trance, when the verbal message might take the form of a 'ventriloquial' direct utterance. If a message formed in the mind of the medium but seemed not to concern the client (or if no client was present) the medium might take it down by some form of 'automatic writing' (Chapter 15). In one interesting case, however, the American housewife Mrs Pearl Curran seemed to have been a medium of sorts, but generally had no clients at all. Her 'controlling spirit' called herself 'Patience Worth' and, using Mrs Curran as operator, wrote a number of books by ouija board, starting in 1913. Worth claimed that she had lived in England in the 1600s and went from there to America, where she was killed by Native American inhabitants. Many of her novels were of such high quality that they were even published. Furthermore, they show remarkable insights into the time about which they were written. Thus one of them, *The Sorry Tale*, was set in Israel in the time of Jesus of Nazareth and displayed great familiarity with the social customs, clothing, commerce and weapons of those times, the topography and architecture of Jerusalem as it was then, and so on. Another, *Telka*, set in medieval England, was composed almost entirely of words of Anglo-Saxon origin. All this appeared far beyond the abilities of Pearl Curran. Sceptical examiners of the output of Patience Worth have claimed that she was just a second personality of Mrs Curran. However, it also makes sense to suppose that Worth was some sort of non-physical being who was using Mrs Curran as a writing instrument.

This is a good example of the many strange phenomena discussed, for example, in Chapters 8 to 11. One of the facts I have had to bear in mind is that psychic power is inherently unpredictable. It comes and goes independently of the human will—a fact which fits my notion that it depends on something outside that will: our unconscious mind. But whatever may cause this unpredictability, it presents the potential medium with a strange but compelling personal problem. Once a medium has brought his or her power to social attention, he or she may frequently be expected to exhibit it on command. Merely to maintain a public position, therefore, a medium can be driven to 'fill in' the gaps by cheating. The inevitable if slow decline of what is in any case a sporadic and unpredictable ability means that a practitioner has to cheat more and more often—and, furthermore, gets better and better at cheating. Indeed, one medium (Eusapia Palladino, in about 1908) cried out to some investigators, 'Hold me tight, or I'll cheat!'—suggesting that dishonesty was already part of her repertoire. I have encountered much the same sort of trickery in television programmes. As transmitted, such a programme has to be totally unambiguous and convincing. To create a 'take' that does this often needs a remarkable degree of trickery 'behind the scenes'. This is often the case if it alleges to show an uncertain phenomenon, or one which can only be done once. To my later shame, I have readily cooperated in setting up such tricks. As I. J. Good remarked, 'A journalist's problem is to get a story. The truth, as such, is not news.' Television producers, journalists and mediums all face this sort of challenge.

In this context, I am reminded of the apocryphal saying 'The difference between the professional and the amateur is that the professional knows when to stop'. In the case of mediums, the professionals are those who do not try to expand their gifts, recognize that such gifts are always uncertain, and will in any case decline with time. I class the true greats in the psychic field as such professionals. Such a one was the medium Daniel Dunglas Home, a Scotsman who lived from 1833 to 1886. Over a career of 25 years as an active medium he was never detected in any fraud.

The founding of the Society for Psychical Research in 1882 and the American one in 1884

In the 1800s, science, and physics in particular, seemed so triumphant that in 1882 the Society for Psychical Research was founded. It aimed to achieve for psychic matters something of what physics had done for material ones. Its first president was Henry Sidgwick. His reputation for sanity, truthfulness and fairness greatly countered the claims of outsiders that the new Society was a collection of fools who solemnly collected the stories of old women and the tricks of imposters. Among its leading luminaries were Frederic Myers and Edmund Gurney. Then, as now, psychic matters and spiritualism were dense with fraud and trickery, but the Society seems to have assumed, almost without considering the problem, that scientific methods should easily detect this. I fear that this is not true. A good trickster will almost always defeat a mere scientist. The Society certainly came across many tricks, but even when it did, many members continued to trust the subject. One scientist even demonstrated that a spirit had breathed out carbon dioxide, yet continued to feel that genuine spiritual encounters were possible.

The Society for Psychical Research has continued as a scientific organization to the present day. Initially it was a British organization, but its American branch soon became independent and published a journal of its own. That American branch suffered many forms of disarray in its early years, but from about 1927 onwards, it achieved great prominence. Its premier laboratory was the Paranormal Laboratory at Duke University, North Carolina, USA, under its leader Joseph Rhine. (It is now independent of the university, and known as the Rhine Research Center.) Perhaps its most interesting discovery was that human beings seem to display a wide spread of something I think of as 'psychic ability'. Human beings differ in many ways: not only height and weight, but also in mental gifts such as scientific insight, creative flair in a field, or psychic ability. The few people with some rare and strange psychic ability are very important to paranormal investigators. In this book I call that subset of those who can guess better than chance, star guessers.

It was in about 1927 that Joseph Rhine started his dramatic work at Duke University, initially under the professor of psychology William McDougall. Joseph and his wife Louisa Rhine essentially set up its famous Parapsychology Laboratory. The couple gave a name to psychic ability: they called it 'Psi' or 'ESP' (for extrasensory perception). They divided it into four sections. 'Telepathy' (a word invented by Frederic Myers) was the ability to know what was in another human mind, without anything being transferred between the minds by speech, writing or other sensory means. 'Clairvoyance' was knowing something which was not present in any human mind at the time. 'Precognition' was the knowledge of something that was currently undecided, but would be established in the future. 'Psychokinesis' was a physical effect: the ability to move or alter an object without touching it or acting on it in any physical way. In 1934 Rhine's book *Extra-Sensory Perception*, which outlined these effects, generated a lot of interest. His basic experiment, which he greatly improved, consisted in asking a guesser to guess which cards were being dealt from a shuffled pack of them. The usual pack of 52 playing cards was not ideal, and Rhine devised a special pack of 'ESP' cards for the job. Zener cards they were called, after their designer Karl Zener.

Rhine supervised a large number of card-guessing experiments (I discuss the matter in Chapter 8 and Appendix B), and on many occasions a card guesser seemed to guess better than one would expect by chance. The resulting publication typically trumpeted this result, together with the absurdly low probability of its having happened by chance, but seldom gave the data and never gave any theory of the finding. In fact even a star guesser exceeded chance only a little (in Appendix B I calculate that a typical excess might be a bit over 7 percent).

Rhine attributed a lot of his success to the invigorating and encouraging atmosphere of his Paranormal Laboratory (Chapter 6). I feel that he was very lucky to find so many star guessers willing to guess for him. Nobody else seems to have managed to replicate his results.

It is worth wondering what sort of unconscious mind a good star guesser might need. I have argued (Chapter 4) that the unconscious mind is inherently a deceiver. It lets very little 'upstairs' to the conscious mind and distorts or disguises anything it does let upstairs. I can imagine three ways in which the unconscious mind of a star guesser might outclass one owned by a normal chance-bound human being. The first is simply to have a sensitive unconscious mind, one that is unusually receptive to promptings from the unknown world. The second might be to have a more forthcoming unconscious mind, one which lets more information 'upstairs'. A third might be to have a more honest unconscious mind, one which distorted the data less in its transmission upstairs. I do not know of any studies on this topic, but I can imagine that the dreams of a star guesser (which must be invented entirely in the unconscious mind) might give useful clues (I discuss dreams in Chapter 10).

Theories about star guessers

I feel emboldened to play with some theories about guessing better than chance. Rhine, perhaps wisely, never did so. Those card-guessing games seem to me to encapsulate a lot of ideas of what may be out in the unknown world beyond our diving bell. Appendix B has some calculations about those who have guessed better than chance. Here I merely note that a 'star' card-guesser never knows when he or she has made a correct guess. I assume that the guess is prompted by something lodged in the unconscious mind and is pushed up into the conscious mind. There the guess is announced and recorded. Presumably it enters the unconscious mind of the star guesser by some sort of telepathy, either from some nearby human mind or from some non-human alien resident in the unknown world. As a catch-all admission of defeat, I include the possibility that it may come from something we know nothing about.

My first option is that key information may come from the past: say from the memories of people who made up the card packs. If those who shuffled and made up the packs never knew what was in them (and they should not have done), they will have known nothing themselves. However, I can imagine that some non-physical entity in the room might have been able to read the cards in a closed pack. 'Feda', the spiritual 'control' of the medium Mrs Gladys Osborne Leonard, once claimed to be able to read a particular page of a book on a bookshelf. Feda did not even need it to be taken down from the shelf and opened at that page. She even claimed to be able to do this for a book that Mrs Leonard herself did not know about. One of Mrs Leonard's clients was a Mrs Talbot, who had in her possession a book in which some words had been written by her dead husband, Hugh. 'Feda' was able to describe the book as a dark leather one about 8 inches by 10 inches, and to quote some of its contents, it began, she said, with a screed about languages. On page 12 or 13 the book had an extract which Feda reckoned that Mrs Talbot should look at. Sure enough, after some searching Mrs Talbot found the book, identified it from

Feda's description, and discovered on page 13 a long extract which the dead Mr Hugh Talbot had copied from an older book, about the situation of someone after death. This is a powerful example of information known to an entity in the unknown world but not to anyone in the physical world. Mrs Leonard tested Feda's abilities on several occasions. Feda sometimes made mistakes, but was often remarkably accurate. This uncanny ability to judge the markings on hidden paper is, of course, exactly the skill we are looking for. If some invisible and unguessed entity in the room could pick up such information from the cards, and convey it unconsciously to the unconscious mind of the guesser, that guesser's ability to guess better than chance would be neatly explained.

My second option is that the information might have come from a human mind in the future. After all, somebody will have had to look at the cards some time after the experiment, so as to be able to judge how well the guesser did. Perhaps that person unconsciously and telepathically transmitted the knowledge back in time to the guesser? It seems impossible for any future knowledge to be transmitted back in time. However, the notion is somewhat supported by studies in which guessers were asked to guess numbers which had not yet been created: they were only generated at some later time—ranging from a few hours to two years. In Chapter 7 I speculate that the unknown world outside our diving bell may have a different sort of time dimensionality to our physical one. If that world is indeed 'outside physical time' it may be able to transmit information back into the past. I recall here that the star card-guesser Basil Shackleton once seemed to be reacting not to present cards, but ones to be presented in three seconds' time. This claim (like many others in parapsychology) has been disputed, but it reminds me of the possible temporal freedom of the unknown world.

My third notion is that the information picked up by the unconscious mind of the card guesser might have come from some non-material entity in the room where the guessing was going on. The room might have contained some non-physical entity which could read the cards, rather as 'Feda' might have done.

My fourth notion is that unlike Feda, who claimed to have been human until her death in about 1800, the entity responsible was never human at all. I include it because I was once inspired by a piece of fiction. The ultimate non-human alien is perhaps the Devil. Arthur Porges's story[31] 'The Devil and Simon Flagg' has the Devil offering to answer any question in return for Flagg's soul. Flagg asks if Fermat's Last Theorem is true. 'Who's last what?' says the Devil, in a hollow voice. He was clearly disconcerted by the challenge. (Fermat discussed his Last Theorem in about 1637. He wrote in the margin of a book: 'I have discovered a truly marvellous proof, which this margin is too narrow to contain.' Over the subsequent centuries, many mathematicians have puzzled over this claim. They all failed to find a proof, and many felt that Fermat had made some mistake. The theorem was finally proved in 1995 by Andrew Wiles, but in 1954 when Porges's story was published, it was one of the most famous unsolved problems in mathematics. The proof, however, does not suggest what Fermat might have set down in that margin, had it been bigger.)

My fifth possibility is indeed an act of defeat, a final catch-all. The information which gets into the mind of a star guesser may simply arrive from some unknown source. Even if it came from the unknown world 'outside our diving bell', we have no idea how it got into a human mind.

15

Getting Information from the Unknown World by Insight and by Writing

In the discussion above I have imagined ways in which a card guesser might do better than chance, essentially by accessing information that reaches his or her unconscious mind. The thesis of this book is that the human unconscious mind is in some sort of weak contact with the unknown world, so that it may occasionally be able to acquire useful information from it. It can then pass it 'upstairs' to the conscious mind, probably distorting it in the process. I imagine that the conscious mind suddenly becomes 'aware' of its new knowledge, but cannot evaluate it and does not know where it came from. Sometimes that conscious mind goes on to 'translate' its new notions into spoken or written language for other people—I have noted a few cases in which the acquisition of new knowledge seems to precede that linguistic translation. In many other

Why Are We Conscious? A Scientist's Take on Consciousness and Extrasensory Perception
David E. H. Jones

ISBN 978-981-4774-32-1 (Hardcover), 978-1-315-16688-9 (eBook)
www.panstanford.com

cases, such as the card-guessing experiments I discuss in the previous chapter, the novel idea remains private. In either case, the unconscious mind is in my view the first information-receiver. Now psychiatrists have put a lot of effort into acquiring data from the unconscious mind. They have explored it in several ways. One is the interpretation of dreams; another is an attempt to get at it slowly via the 'talking cure'. Either way, the psychiatrist hopes to explore memories or aspects of the personality of the patient which have been 'repressed' into the unconscious mind. I do not know why this recovery is beneficial to the patient, but it often is. I assume that most of the data in the patient's unconscious mind is not disturbed by this enquiry; indeed, the psychiatrist usually has no idea what might be there. Here I want to talk not about notions from the conscious mind pushed into the unconscious one by repression, but about ways in which the unconscious mind can acquire information from the unknown world, which it can then pass 'upstairs' into consciousness. The first way is extremely rare and valuable. I call it 'insight'.

Insight

Insight is simply having an idea. It seems just to emerge in the conscious mind. My feeling is that it must have got there from the unconscious one. Many 'seers' have such insights. Often they are predictions or divinations of the distant future. Predictions about the future assume (Chapter 7) that the unknown world is somehow 'outside time'. If so, the future already exists for it, and it can pass information about the future back to the unconscious mind of the seer. Once the unconscious mind of a seer acquires knowledge of some future event, that knowledge is then sent 'upstairs' to the conscious mind, where it appears as a prediction. One of the most famous of modern seers was the blind Bulgarian Vanga Dimitrova. Often a client only had to come into her presence to trigger a set of insights. Thus she might use a 'pet name' only known to the members of that person's family or might describe correctly personal details about past or present marriages or relationships that only that person would know. She might even predict a date or mode of death for that person or a relative, perhaps many years in the future.

Some of her insights were encouragingly positive. Thus a client sometimes came to ask her about someone they feared for, and Vanga was able to tell that client that the individual was still alive, was currently engaged in some specified activity, and that they would meet again in stated circumstances.

In 1966 Vanga Dimitrova was adopted by the Bulgarian government to be the central figure in the newly established scientific research Institute of Suggestology and Parapsychology in Sofia and Petrich (the village in which she lived). That Institute reckoned that her predictions were about 80 percent correct—which makes me suspect that even for a seer, the unconscious mind often defends its data by distorting it a bit before passing it 'upstairs'. Vanga said that she had no control over the images that formed in her 'mind's eye'. She could not force them and did not know where they came from. She lost her sight as a teenager (it might have been saved if her family could have afforded an expensive medical procedure), and I now wonder if its loss increased her paranormal powers. It is frequently the case that losing one sense makes the others more acute.

Vanga Dimitrova must certainly be counted among my successful mediums. The mediums who flourished during World War I, claiming to provide bereaved survivors with a message from a deceased person, were more dubious. Kipling's disturbing poem 'En-dor' may reflect an attempt of his to make contact with his own son, who died in that war. Thomas Huxley denounced the whole business of obtaining messages from the dead and said that it merely provided an extra argument against suicide. Conversely, Arthur Conan Doyle, he of the Sherlock Holmes stories, was a great believer in transmissions from 'the other side'. He once claimed to have received some sentences from the shade of Oscar Wilde. Many aphorisms from Oscar Wilde, such as 'Vulgarity is the rich man's modest contribution to democracy', have been recorded in the publications of the self-proclaimed medium Hester Travers Smith. That arch sceptic the biologist J. B. S. Haldane denounced such claims. 'Death certainly had a bad effect on Wilde's genius,' he remarked.

An extreme sort of insight may be that type of impulse called 'enlightenment'. Sometimes, as with Gautama Buddha, the enlightened person goes on to found a religion. Sometimes, as with Descartes, it simply has a transformative personal effect. Aldous Huxley has discussed the dramatic impact that it can bring about, and that it has inspired many people to become the leaders of movements or cults. I do not understand this sort of insight, but accept that it may have a component which comes from the unknown world. Stanislav Grof (Chapter 8) has identified two types, the 'oceanic' and the 'volcanic' forms. He reckons that we may all potentially carry them: they relate to the universal memory of being in the womb, and later of being born. Against this notion, many physiologists have claimed that our nervous system, which governs the sort of memories we can form, is still very undeveloped even at birth. I imagine that a baby may form inter-uterine memories, but do not know if they can later be elaborated. I have read, for example, that a foetus can hear the mother's heartbeat in the womb, so that a baby can often be calmed by hearing a recording of such a beat–it makes the baby think of the comfort of foetal existence. I also recall that some expectant mothers wear a loudspeaker system by which specific music, or specific words, are played to the foetus in the womb, with the idea of affecting its later tastes or getting its knowledge off to a good start. My feeling is that while such systems may have some useful effect, early memories are generally very limited. I suppose that they may help to determine later musical taste, but doubt that they can play a significant part in the process known as 'enlightenment'.

Spirit writing

A popular component of many Victorian séances was 'spirit writing' on a slate. A slate which was originally blank was later found to have writing on it, allegedly a message from some unknown world. In the same way, a piece of paper could apparently receive a message written on it by a pencil. Lord Rayleigh once put a pencil and a piece of paper in a glass vessel, pumped it down to vacuum to prevent trickery, and left it for years to see if any writing would appear on the paper. He later found that 'the opportunity appears to have been neglected'. If any writing had appeared on his paper, Lord Rayleigh might have shown it to a graphologist. With luck the graphologist would have helped to identify the author: perhaps somebody who had recently died. I have suggested (Chapter 9) that the incoherent actions of poltergeists are not due to jokiness or annoyance, but simply due to clumsiness. Accordingly, now that manual writing has largely been replaced by key-pressing, I can imagine a new version of Lord Rayleigh's experiment. The pencil might be replaced by a keyboard of very large or widely spaced keys. Even a very clumsy entity could then spell out a message on that keyboard. Lord Rayleigh would have needed a very large glass container to enclose such an apparatus and to pump it down to an effective vacuum.

I am inclined to disregard stories of spirit writing. If genuine, the writing should have been the wild useless scribble one might expect from a clumsy poltergeist. This implies that the usual neat writing was probably fraudulent. Indeed, I know of no message that seems genuine. In the absence of good examples or any suggestive evidence, I shall just dismiss the technique altogether. I recall, however, that it dates back to the Old Testament biblical story about the writing on the wall (Daniel, Chapter 5, verse 25) and that several artists, including Rembrandt, have depicted the scene.

Automatic writing

In automatic writing, the arm and hand are encouraged to move under unconscious control. They push a pencil over a blank sheet of paper, but the conscious mind makes no attempt to impose anything on the writing. The resulting script is then the product of the unconscious mind and possibly comes from the unknown world. Automatic writing in its various forms is as questionable as data obtained in any other way. It seems, however, to have recorded by far the greatest amount of information of any technique. Two items of technology have been widely used: the planchette and the ouija board. The planchette is a small trolley, with two castor wheels. The third supporting member is a pencil. The operator just pushes it over a piece of paper without attempting to impose anything on its movement. The planchette sometimes produces a sequence of letters which can be interpreted as a written script. I have mused that one of its useful effects may be to restrain the wild attempts of an arm without physical skill to control a pencil.

The ouija board is even simpler. It is a board with (for example) the letters of the alphabet on it, and the mathematical numerals. You push an indicator around the board to pick out the symbol you plan to use next. It was invented in China around the 1000s. I imagine that the huge number of characters in written Chinese, and the difficulty of delineating any one of them with a brush, meant that the board greatly simplified the task of writing Chinese. In the late 1800s the ouija board appeared in an English version. It was widely sold as a toy, but it also seems to have been used by authors as a way of jogging their inventiveness, thus breaking 'writer's block'. Both devices remove the need for a writer to show any physical skill. Later, both devices acquired spiritualistic significance.

The planchette and the ouija board have been used many times in an attempt to obtain messages from some unknown world. A practised medium may be able to distract the conscious mind almost at will, so as to generate by 'automatic writing' a script that may have come from the unconscious mind. He or she may be asked by a client to receive a message from someone 'on the other side'. But if the medium feels that a message of some sort is coming in, but is not addressed to an immediate client, that medium may acquire and take down that message by 'automatic writing', using a variant of one of the methods I am discussing here.

An interesting outcome of the creation of the Society for Psychical Research was that one of its main founders, Frederic Myers, published a brave book about death. It was titled *Human Personality and Its Survival of Bodily Death* and came out in 1903, two years after Myers's death, in 1901. He once claimed that after his own death his ghost would act so forcefully that survival after death could not be doubted. In the event, his ghost seems not to have haunted anybody, but after death he seems to have cooperated with two other dead members of the Society. They sent messages back to the living world by automatic writing. The entities who seem to have cooperated in this venture were Edmund Gurney (who died in 1888) and Henry Sidgwick (who died in 1900). All three had been classical scholars. These post-death entities seemed aware of many problems facing a joint transmission, and invented a clever 'cross-correspondence' system to transfer information to the physical world, and to assure that world of its authenticity. The basic notion was to send messages to each of several mediums not known to each other, by 'automatic writing'. Thus at one point the shade of Myers, in a message to Alice Johnson, then the secretary of the Society for Psychical Research, encouraged Miss Johnson in her automatic writing. She wrote, 'My hand feels very shaky; shall I just let it scrawl?' And the shade replied, 'Yes, let it go quite freely, just exactly as it likes!' Each message itself would mean nothing, but a proper combination of the three would make sense. All three men had been classical scholars. Each of their cross-correspondences was dense with classical allusions; I imagine that this was intended both to baffle the mediums and to identify the authors. The mediums they chose seem to have included Mrs W. de G. Verrall and her daughter Helen Verrall, who were classical scholars themselves. They also included Mrs L. E. Piper, 'Mrs Willett' (Mrs Winifred Coombe-Tennant) and Mrs Holland (the sister of Rudyard Kipling), who were not.

Many messages were picked up by the chosen mediums, and appear to have verified that Myers, Gurney and Sidgwick had survived death. Indeed, they seem to have retained enough knowledge and intellectual power to compose and send the messages. The many cross-correspondences received by the mediums were published in several issues of the Proceedings of the Society for

Psychical Research between about 1903 and 1930. They were made into several books, notably H. F. Saltmarsh's publication of 1938, *Evidence of Personal Survival from Cross Correspondences*. However, they may have been deformed in transmission, for they resisted full decoding into a clear summed statement. Many of the messages received by the mediums contained complaints from their apparent authors 'on the other side'. It seems that they had great difficulty transmitting a message to the physical world. Thus the shade of Myers complained at one point, 'There is so much to say, and yet so very little chance of saying it—communication is so tremendously difficult—the brain of the agent [i.e. the automatic writer] though indispensable is so hampering!' Myers and others had great trouble even in establishing their identities, let alone getting across their joint message. Again, Myers deplored the trouble of saying anything: 'The nearest simile I can find to express the difficulties of sending a message is that I appear to be standing behind a sheet of frosted glass—which blurs sight and deadens sound—dictating feebly to a reluctant and somewhat obtuse secretary. A feeling of terrible impotence burdens me . . .'

There are many examples, real or fake, of messages apparently sent from dead persons to living ones. It interests me that in another case of apparent transmission from someone dead, the wrong identity came through. In 1930, the medium Eileen Garrett set up a séance in the hope of interviewing the recently dead Sir Arthur Conan Doyle. She found herself talking to the spirit of Flight Lieutenant Carmichael Irwin, captain of the recently lost R101 airship. She maintained the exchange and obtained information about the poor design of the R101, and some reasons for its crash.

My impression is that the unknown world is very weakly coupled to the material one. Even if among its inhabitants it contains entities which retain some aspects of people now dead, it is very hard to transmit an intelligible message from it to an unconscious mind in the physical world. The same sort of problem often occurs in another mental transmission, that of telepathy (Chapter 8). I suspect that the unconscious mind adds to this problem by habitually distorting or disguising anything it 'lets upstairs' to consciousness (Chapter 4). Later (Chapter 16) I suggest that a computer specially intended to communicate with the unknown world might do better.

Perhaps the most successful attempt to obtain information from the unknown world by automatic writing was that of Frederick Bond and John Alleyne in the early 1900s. Bond later wrote a book, *The Gate of Remembrance*,[5] about their experience. They were both interested in Glastonbury Abbey, a fine building destroyed in 1539 by Henry VIII in his dissolution of the monasteries. The magnificence of the building was such that John Leland, 'King's antiquary' to Henry VIII, was moved by awe when he looked at it, and perhaps even Henry VIII was unhappy to destroy it. In about 1900 the owner of the site was the Church of England. It decided to recreate some of the lost Abbey and chose Bond as a major project architect. Bond reckoned that the buried foundations of the lost building would be a very good start if he could find them. He was a member of the Society of Psychical Research, and Alleyne had had previous experience of psychic automatism. The two men decided to see if spiritualism could help. Both of them knew Everard Feilding, the secretary of the Society, who maintained much interest in the work and made many helpful suggestions. They began to seek out long-dead Glastonbury monks by automatic writing. Their method was simple but effective. Alleyne held a pencil over a large sheet of paper, and Bond laid his hand on the back of Alleyne's hand. Alleyne's hand, with Bond's hand on top of it, did the actual automatic writing. The pair then started a session, which Bond initiated by asking a question verbally, as if addressing someone else in the room. Whatever entity might reply could either hear his spoken words or react to the thought in his mind. Indeed, on one occasion Bond asked a question purely mentally, without speaking, and got a reply. I suspect that an entity in the unknown world may be able to read a thought in a conscious mind before it gets translated into language. Anyway, Bond's question often initiated a session of automatic writing, sometimes with drawn plans. During the session the two receiving men maintained a friendly but relaxed and distracting dialogue: one practice was for Bond to read aloud to Alleyne from some entertaining book. When one piece of paper was full of script or drawing, Alleyne got a clean sheet, and the session continued.

The pencil in Alleyne's hand, seemingly automatically, often traced out plans of unsuspected buried details, and writings apparently from some of the long-dead men who had known the building in its days of glory. Among this 'Company of Glaston' was Abbot Beere, a great builder who constructed several extensions around 1500. Some of the automatic writing obtained by Bond and Alleyne seemed to come from the long-dead Abbot himself. Thus one passage, received on 16 June 1908, about the dimensions in feet of the then unknown Edgar chapel, went, 'The width ye shall find is seven and twenty, and outside thirty and four, so we remember—beere abbas.' Bond and Alleyne seem to have made contact with several other dead people, including 'Johannes de Glaston', who is not otherwise known to history. Bond's initial question might be directly answered in the writing. Alternatively, the writing might deal with quite another matter. The lapse of time seemed not to exist for it. Thus it might take up a discussion which had been discontinued some days or even months previously. Bond felt that their technique was related to the 'gift of tongues' mentioned in the Christian Bible. Thus he quotes a letter from St. Paul (Corinthians 1, Chapter 14), in which the recipient of the 'gift of tongues' does not know what he or she is saying. Indeed, the 'automatic writings' recorded on the paper often puzzled the two receivers by being written in a strange mixture of Low Latin, Middle English of various periods and Modern English in differing styles and dictions. The 'hand' of the writing could change too, as if a different entity had taken over from the previous one. Sessions were limited in time, perhaps typically half an hour to an hour. Towards the end of a session the writing was often weaker and fainter, as if fatigue were setting in, but it is hard to decide whether that fatigue was human or from the unknown origin of the writing. Bond and Alleyne conducted over a hundred sessions between 1907 and 1918, mainly in the first few years.

Quite apart from the mixture of languages and styles, the two receivers had much trouble deciphering the automatic script. The entity responsible for the writing often complained that the material influences were wrong, or other influences were crossing his own. Bond felt like a man on the telephone, with the operator always switching him into other conversations, or with the wiring so badly insulated that they could obtrude anyway. It was not obvious whether he was conversing with a specific personality, or with a larger field of memory to which human recollections contributed. This example is probably the best instance we have of information obtained by automatic writing. In due course the Church of England discovered from Bond's book that it had been inadvertently involved in spiritualism. It sacked Bond and withdrew all support for him. Even so, Glastonbury is now a major artistic and theological centre.

Bond comments that while he got much useful information about the Edgar Chapel at Glastonbury, his questions about the Loretto Chapel got nowhere. Such information that he did receive bore no useful relation to what he was able to discover by digging at the site. I am inclined to suspect that, assuming automatic writing gets into the unconscious mind, which drives the hand and arm of the human writer, it is always liable to be distorted almost automatically by that unconscious mind. You might therefore almost expect that any message received by automatic writing will be inaccurate in some way. This is also perhaps why the clever cross-correspondences of Myers, Gurney and Sidgwick did not combine properly into their intended total message.

Bond's story is remarkably echoed in a novel of 1948, *No Highway*, by Nevil Shute (I have mentioned it in Chapter 10). Mr Honey, Shute's central character, refers to Glastonbury several times. He also talks about his experience of asking souls 'on the other side' to describe architectural structures now destroyed, so as to verify their replies by digging. Honey employs his adolescent daughter to operate a planchette in his search for a missing aircraft component. I suspect that Shute had read Bond's book and knew some of the themes in it.

16

Getting Information from the Unknown World

IS THERE ANY WAY OF MAKING CONTACT with the unknown world outside our diving-bell? I have never found any scientific or instrumental way into it. That world only seems to make contact with a few human unconscious minds, and then only occasionally. Sceptics can deny its existence with complete impunity. But if it exists, there should be some way of demonstrating that fact, and I like the idea of looking for it scientifically. In Chapter 7 I imagine a way of showing its existence by small thermal effects. It seems to have many abilities: not least those of creating actions in the physical world (as in the various forms of psychokinesis, some of which I discuss in Chapter 9). Yet it is probably best to think of it as a source of information. Sometimes, as in many types of telepathy, that information is so direct and transparent that the receiver has taken it as a true sensory impression. At other times, as in many dreams (Chapter 10) the

Why Are We Conscious? A Scientist's Take on Consciousness and Extrasensory Perception
David E. H. Jones

ISBN 978-981-4774-32-1 (Hardcover), 978-1-315-16688-9 (eBook)
www.panstanford.com

information is so strongly disguised that it needs some sort of interpretation. I fear that such disguise is usual. The unconscious human mind is so inherently deceptive that most communications that it allows 'upstairs' need to be interpreted or decoded in some way, and this may warn us that equivalent deception may occur in the transfer of information from the unknown world to the unconscious mind. I was greatly touched by the description given by the dead Myers (whom I discuss in Chapter 15) of the frustration he felt in his attempts to communicate from the unknown world to the physical living one. He may, of course, have been part of some entity in the unknown world, but his written complaint seems like one from a single individual. He felt greatly hampered by having to deal with the brain of the person he was trying to send a message to, though he felt that brain contact was indispensable. He even had great difficulty in just sending his identity to that brain. I assume that his message was initially aimed at the unconscious mind of the receiver, who would then have the troublesome or even uncontrollable hand-and-arm task of writing it out by automatic writing. The process might have been much easier if it had been conducted not by a rare and unreliable human being, but by some fast machine. At present the only way of making any contact with that unknown world is via the highly uncertain and baffling human unconscious mind, but I am reminded of the early days of current electricity. It could be observed by the way it made a pair of freshly dissected frog's legs twitch. Much later, electrical instruments were devised which did not depend on a special preparation of once-living material. In the same sort of way, we may initially find that we have to exploit the abilities of a few rare gifted living individuals, but the advance of experimental methods might ultimately allow us to make useful contact with the world outside our diving bell by constructed inorganic instrumentation. I cannot guess how or in what way this might happen: but it would be a wonderful advance. My guesses below continues my feelings about moving research into the unconscious mind away from the mysteries of living systems to the more controllable inorganic ones used by instrument makers. Those guesses include my musings on the experiments with bacterial cultures that inspired Alexander Fleming to invent penicillin.

One great advantage of any scientific instrument which could access the unknown world would to bring that world out of the shadowy 'paranormal' field and into the certain world of physical science. Instead of depending on the changing and unpredictable states of mind of individual observers, it would enter the Valérian world of believable, repeatable, scientific observations—the recipes which always work. Great speed would be an advantage too. The automatic writing project of Bond and Alleyne, for example (Chapter 15), took about ten years. I like the idea of replacing their crude, slow, hand-based automatic writing by modern fast electronic processing and text printing. Another story of slow automatic writing concerns a British soldier in South Africa about 1900, killed by a bullet though his spine. In that sudden and final distress, he seems to have sent a message to his sister about 6000 miles away in London. It describes his sudden plight, gives the names of the comrades who helped him in his last moments, and asks for them to be given certain keepsakes from his property.

Computer-based interrogation

In Chapter 4 I expound a notion of the unconscious mind. I claim that to be conscious at all you have to have one, and that is why no computer can be conscious. Even so, I like the idea of encouraging research into computer-based artificial intelligence (AI) in that direction. All practical computers these days have the 'von Neumann architecture' espoused by the great computer pioneer John von Neumann. In this design, many memory cells each hold a number. Each step in the computer program requires the central processor to take a copy of the number in each of one or more specified cells, perform some mathematical operation on its take, and deliver the results to specific other cells. Several attempts have been made to devise a different 'non-von' architecture. They may include the current attempts to devise a 'quantum computer'. Could such a computer be given have an unconscious mind? I do not know, but I like the idea.

As before, I allow myself to be inspired by fiction. One character in Arthur C. Clarke's famous novel[8] *2001: A Space Odyssey* was the conscious computer HAL. HAL was not built so much as grown, by a process rather like the growth of a human brain. Nowhere was there any set of circuit diagrams and nobody knew at all how HAL worked. Nonetheless, the growth process resulted in a machine which convinced its operators, the astronauts David Bowman and Frank Poole, that they were dealing with a conscious intelligence. HAL would have fitted neatly into my ideas about a conscious computer with an unconscious mind. Indeed, HAL had a psychiatric breakdown (suggesting that he did indeed have an unconscious mind) and showed fear when Bowman had to kill him.

Exploring life other than the human variety

A second notion of mine is that the unknown world seems to make contact only with living organisms. Life, consciousness and the unconscious mind are still beyond any sort of scientific theory. At present, there seems no reason why any object made of atoms can be conscious. There isn't even a test for consciousness: the question I pose in Chapter 1—'Is a beetle conscious?'—simply cannot be answered. The only conscious things we know about are life forms, notably human beings and the higher animals. All of them have a biochemistry based on carbon. The 'intelligent aliens' that H. G. Wells imagined in his *War of the Worlds* of 1898, and that astronomers and others have pondered ever since, might not have such a chemistry: their chemistry might be entirely different and might not matter anyway. So one way forward might be to look for some interaction of the unknown world with living systems. Such a way is the culturing of cells in a Petri dish, in a suitable nutrient medium. Alexander Fleming recognized penicillin by making a contaminated culture; he did not just throw it away, but studied it and saw in it a new medical direction. So maybe there is some sort of interaction between a cell culture and the unknown world. Indeed, professional culture-makers may be already being familiar with it. They conventionally grow their cultures in agar jelly. It may well be true that agar is the best jelly former for general bacterial work. Yet there must be dozens of other jelly-forming substances, and some other, more restricted one may hold the clue we need. It may, of course, require the enquiring mind of an Alexander Fleming to spot and try it.

Liquid theory

Another possible approach grows out of my dissatisfaction with liquid theory. The liquid state has a character of its own—for example, it encompasses nearly all chemistry. Life, and *a fortiori* consciousness, occurs only in the liquid phase. All biological cells contain not merely liquid water and many substances in solution, but lots of objects in aqueous suspension as well. Astronomers searching for a planet which might support extraterrestrial life (and to date they have not found one) concentrate on planets whose surface temperature is compatible with the existence of water as a liquid. There may be subtle wisdom in the way that many computer experts call the human brain's mental contribution to a computer program, one from 'wetware'.

If liquid molecules can carry information, some of it may be impressed on them from the unknown world. Existing physical theory regards their orientation and movement as entirely random and bearing no information. This may be true for gases, as shown by the brilliant success of Maxwell's kinetic theory of gases. His theory has been pretty much taken over for liquids too. Current theory imagines liquid molecules moving and tumbling in a pure random 'drunkard's walk'. This assumption fits the observed bulk property of a liquid, and also the Brownian motion of fine suspended particles. Brownian motion is allegedly caused by the random way in which suspended particles get hit by liquid molecules. It was brilliantly used by Perrin in his classic experiments on molecular theory. And yet Boris Derjaguin,[12] the discoverer of 'polywater', was intrigued to find that the molecules of a liquid (and he tried several liquids other than water: benzene, for example) could be greatly influenced by the information carried by a solid surface. Polywater was ultimately rejected by the chemical community. It could only be obtained in extremely fine capillary tubes. By contrast, an accepted new substance such as heavy water could be made in bucketsful. Nonetheless, this book is essentially about concealed information, so I am interested in the idea that the molecules of a liquid might somehow contain information. They may do so by their spin. This seems to have been ignored in liquid theory—indeed I know of only one scientific paper which comments on spin in molecules of a liquid.

In Chapter 11 I discuss the way that the biochemist Jacques Benveniste upset himself and the editor of *Nature*, John Maddox. Benveniste found that his solvent, water, appeared to carry information, and suspected that it might somehow 'remember' the molecules which had once been dissolved in it. There are several ways in which the information in a liquid—if it has any—can get amplified up for observation. Some forms of spectroscopy may do this, and so may 'critical opalescence'. A pressurized liquid being converted into a gas of the same density shows, for a specific narrow temperature range, a scattering of transmitted light due to its variations of density. When those variations have the same sort of size as a wavelength of light, we can see them. So the study of critical opalescence might reveal some way in which a liquid could carry information from the unknown world.

An even weaker search for some way of detecting the unknown world would simply be undirected experiments of any kind. This is not just a counsel of despair; it is inspired by memories of my own research career. Many times as an experimenter, I tried things out with some completely wrong theory in my head and learned from the unexpected results. Mother Nature is always much cleverer than the investigator! Most scientific instruments are either elaborations of human senses (such as the telescope and the microscope) or ways of registering very small forces (such as the balance, and the meters which register the force of an electrical current in a magnetic field). So it may be that the unknown world is detectable by some very simple experiment using a new instrument, although the researcher could be looking for something else.

Decryption

These ideas about detecting the unknown world are mere suggestions for research that might be done. They are probably all wrong, but I still feel that the trick, or even several tricks, is worth some work. However, even if information from the unknown world can be grabbed and turned into something physical, we are only half-way there. Suppose, for example, that such information can be got into some non-von computer's 'unconscious mind'. There are many examples in this book of unconscious minds which strongly resist letting data 'upstairs' into the conscious mind, unless the data is coded to defeat that conscious mind. Thus, in Chapter 10, I give an example from my own stroke, in which a true observation was mentally elaborated or coded into a completely false and fantastic development.

What might we be able to do about by clever distortion or disguise, apart from looking out for it? Effective deception will not merely take the form of contaminating the message by adding meaningless random garbage. It will probably be very subtly and cunningly distorted on its way 'upstairs'. Both my account of Elias Howe's dream in Chapter 4 and my own stroke experience of fantasies elaborated from real observation in Chapter 10 imply that it might be based on mental prior knowledge and not on mathematics at all. Even very clever programming might get nowhere with it. And yet the sort of cleverness we may need is advancing rapidly. The current leaders in decryption may be government spying agencies, such as such as the American NSA, the British GCHQ and the Israeli Mossad. The British agency HM Revenue and Customs, which has to handle many false tax-returns, may also have a computer program to detect and correct deception. Private industry also has decryption skills which we may be able to exploit and develop for new tasks. Google (for example) uses a huge computer algorithm to handle and order a vast amount of conflicting information of all types.

The only clue I can offer is the human hand. Both automatic writing (Chapter 15) and the strange skill of dowsing (Chapter 11) seem to imply that the human unconscious mind has some special connection with the hand. This fits with the curious and powerful way that in automatic writing, the hand seems to be driven directly by the unconscious mind. The human hand is, of course, a recently evolved organ. It has been credited with many of the mighty advances that human beings have made over all other animals. The hand that 'fringed polyp, the best servant that ever could be', has been applauded for launching 'Homo Faber', the tool maker and tool user who has conquered almost all the globe. The motor cortex of the human brain has a huge section devoted to controlling the hand, and a search for clues in this part of the brain cortex might well be worthwhile. George Orwell once wrote, 'Cease to use your hands, and you have chopped off a huge chunk of your consciousness.' I suspect that you have also chopped off a huge chunk of your unconsciousness.

So even though deception and fantasy are probably inevitable, it may be possible to correct much of it electronically. I am encouraged by the success of the first electronic computer in the world, the vacuum-tube monster Colossus of the 1940s. It was built by a British team at Bletchley Park to help crack the German 'Enigma' military codes of World War II, and I once had the honour of talking to its chief designer, Tommy Flowers of the Post Office. He came to Newcastle University in 1977 to receive a richly deserved honorary degree. Many of the radio interceptions of the Enigma code were indeed usefully decoded by Colossus. The decoding power of computers has advanced enormously since those early days, and I suspect that a useful amount of decoding may be made quite automatic. An effective decoding computer program will, of course, have to be familiar with the knowledge which a mind may possess, and the games which an unconscious mind is likely to play.

Even so, a final human scan could well be worthwhile. I have read, for example, that in the 1970s the oil company Standard Oil of New Jersey was looking for a new trademark. 'Esso' had been known for much of the 1900s, a new name seemed desirable. One company approach was to generate names at random by a computer program, and let a human publicist scan the results. In one run the computer programmer had, quite understandably, omitted to warn the randomizing program that in English you are not allowed to put two x's together, and among its output was the suggested name 'Exxon'. The human publicist spotted its value, and the company chose the name. This sort of insightful human skill may not be far from the form of interpretation by which a psychiatrist deduces the 'latent content' of a dream from the 'manifest content' relayed to him by the patient. Lord Adrian has already described one psychiatric procedure as 'outwitting the unconscious'.

Information we might look for

What sort of information should we look for in the unknown world? I like the idea of proving that the information is indeed from some outside source, by seeking things unknown to any existing human mind. Thus we might try to obtain the ten-billionth digit of pi, or the fine-structure constant to twelve decimal places, purely as a powerful way of convincing sceptics that a new source of information does indeed exist. Another form of information would be a proof of the mathematical 'Goldbach conjecture', that every even number is the sum of two prime numbers. It would be equally pleasing to have a counter-example, an even number that is not the sum of two prime numbers. Still, on the subject of mathematics, many modern codes are based on 'trap-door functions' that can go easily one way, but are very hard to reverse. Thus it is quite easy to multiply two hundred-digit numbers together to get a two-hundred-digit number. It is very hard to decide whether a two-hundred-digit number can be obtained by multiplying two hundred-digit numbers together, and to determine what those numbers are. A method of decomposing a big number into smaller ones, as well as being a great mathematical advance, would be worth many millions. It would threaten a vast number of secret codes!

Another dream of mine is that of recovering lost historical information. This dream proposes a positive answer to the poetic question posed by John Donne: 'Tell me where all past years are.' Let us imagine that they exist somewhere in the unknown world. Indeed, if that world is 'outside time', data from both the past and the future should exist in it (Chapter 7). It seems feasible to dream that we might be able to access information both from the future and from the past.

An example of past information might be to restore one of the most tragic events in recorded history. Around 48 BC the Great Library of Alexandria was burnt down. Huge quantities of precious documents were destroyed. My hope is that that library still somehow exists in the past, in the unknown world. How splendid it would be if Feda (who could read a closed book; Chapter 14), or some other entity we might have some control over, could be persuaded to read them and tell us about them! Reading those books before their destruction would give us a vast number of insights into the ancient world.

A more modern exploration would be to look at the increasing numbers of mechanically generated recordings which now cannot be retrieved because the technology has changed. NASA, for example, has had to mount a search for old tape-recorders capable of playing the tapes recorded from early satellite transmissions. Indeed, analog tape recording has been entirely replaced by digital coding. I can easily imagine that as technology advances and new coding methods develop, each will leave behind a huge collection of unplayable records. I can imagine that you might be able to present the machine not with a closed book but with a floppy disk and read it without playing it. Again, a vast amount of hidden information might be recovered.

17

Some Technical Questions for the Unknown World

Trying to acquire new information from the unknown world is not the only way in which we might exploit its riches. Another would be to ask it practical questions about things we cannot do. It might give our technology a huge boost. Again, I cannot imagine what might be available. My first instinct would be to ask questions about the sort of technology of which glimpses have already emerged in the physical world. All our technology assumes that every material has a set of stable properties, essentially set by the forces between its atoms. Accordingly, instances in which they appear to alter briefly (as in Chapter 11) seem very puzzling to us. Thus, one of the tricks which we might want to know more about is some way of bending metals easily. 'Spoon bending', for example, which has both been shown on television and denounced as trickery, would be a very clever way of bending metal if it could be made repeatable and reliable. At present it is neither.

Why Are We Conscious? A Scientist's Take on Consciousness and Extrasensory Perception
David E. H. Jones

ISBN 978-981-4774-32-1 (Hardcover), 978-1-315-16688-9 (eBook)
www.panstanford.com

Nobody in the metal-forming business is worried that it might be developed into something to replace industrial presses, forges and the like. Similarly wood, a rigid material used in so many beams and much furniture, has been made psychically flexible enough for tables to be able to waltz around on their legs. I speculate that this may be part of some wider phenomenon whereby the physical properties of many systems may be briefly and usefully altered. At present we know nothing about this; most substances most of the time seem to have entirely stable properties. If they can be changed at all, they need alterations of temperature, applications of force, or chemical treatment. My speculations that healing and homoeopathy are ultimately due to brief changes in the properties of water, are just that—speculations. Similarly, I am interested in that Russian claim to have communicated with a submerged military submarine by animal telepathy (Chapter 8). Once again, to be useful any technique has to be given some sort of procedure which makes it repeatable and reliable—which at present telepathy certainly is not.

A technical-minded enquirer can easily imagine huge numbers of questions of this sort which might be worth exploring. The field is vast, quite unmapped, and my own guesses are no better than those of anyone else. I can imagine that advances in our understanding of the unknown world, if it exists, could lead to even more dramatic technical achievements. I have already mused (Chapter 7) about the dream of using the cold of that world as a condenser to solve our problems with generating energy. Another scheme which intrigues me is a way of making huge diamonds. They are only carbon, but imagine a diamond weighing (say) a kilogram, materialised from the unknown world, or made under directions from it. It would shatter our whole financial system! It would also make possible all sorts of new technical devices—diamond windows and cells and prisms for spectrometers, diamond heat-sinks to transform computers, even diamond fibre to revolutionize engineering.

It would also be interesting to find out, maybe by studies of future technology, whether the current craze for nanotechnology will get anywhere. When (to my and many other people's dismay) the University of Newcastle upon Tyne closed its physics department, one successor was a nanotechnology department. One media organization has ordered its writers to ignore all scientific progress except in five areas, of which one is nanotechnology. Eric Drexler, a great advocate of this field, has imagined 'assemblers' about the size of bacteria, which can build anything by the manipulation of single atoms. A favourite material of his is carbon. A structure built as he imagines it would be essentially diamond. And yet the only nanotechnological, or even microtechnological, progress that I know of is the making of ever-smaller circuits for computers and electronic gadgets by the optically defined etching of tiny silicon elements.

Perhaps the most dramatic change resulting from information gained from the unknown world would be in space travel. At the moment, the huge physical distances between stars seem to make it impossible for us ever to meet alien life forms, even if they exist. Schemes have already been tried by which we hope to communicate with aliens via radio, or receive their own signals (no successes either way have been reported). One powerful genre of science fiction requires aliens and humans to meet and interact. Writers in this genre have been forced to invent various technical ploys for traversing enormous distances. Arthur C. Clarke has imagined a 'transfinite drive' which allows a space ship to travel around the galaxy. One might expect there to be many non-human 'aliens', some possessed of superhuman knowledge and technical power. And yet the aliens, by whom many people have claimed to have been abducted, have almost universally come to earth in vehicles which simply traverse space, typically 'flying saucers'.

My suspicion is that really advanced aliens might not have to bother at all with the dreary and time-consuming business of space travel. They might be able to get to anywhere that interests them directly, via the unknown world. I was once told of a hospital patient who was confined to bed and could only look out of a window onto the street. He saw people passing the hospital. He decided to call a man a 'dot', a woman a 'dash', and to see what sort of message the passing pedestrians built up in Morse code. Soon he got the message 'You are being watched'. This story interests me. It suggests aliens are already here. Indeed, they may be influencing human society by affecting the decisions that people make all the time, for example, as they walk. I do not take this story very seriously. It is, perhaps, yet another example of my ready use of fiction when facts elude me. And yet it also reminds me of a joke which the great physicist Enrico Fermi made when he was discussing the way that there should be lots of aliens, yet they contrive to remain elusive. Jokingly he said, 'They are already here. And they call themselves Hungarian.' He was perhaps thinking of Albert Szent-Györgyi, Leo Szilard, Dennis Gabor, Eugene Wigner, John von Neumann, and Edward Teller, all brilliant Hungarian scientists. All born around 1900, they greatly advanced their chosen fields.

The unknown world outside our diving bell might make it feasible to make real contact with aliens and learn something about their beliefs and their way of life. They, of course, would learn a lot about ours as well. Even if aliens are very rare, I like the idea of being able to abandon the expensive and difficult technologies of conventional rocket travel. I dream of just entering the unknown world somewhere and exiting it again many light-years away in physical space, without all that tedious physical travelling.

18

Concluding Remarks

My text looks critically at some huge gaps in our scientific knowledge. I often suggest observations which might be made or directions in which research might go. As a retired chemical researcher, I am discomfited by the many things we do not know. (Thus I applaud the great success of atomic theory in accounting for the properties and behaviour of so many substances. Yet cosmologists, as I explain in Chapter 2, now feel that much of the universe is not atomic at all, but 'dark matter'. Where and what is it? My inexpert guess is that if it exists, it does so as dense clumps or nuclei in the centres of stars or planets, so that surface creatures like ourselves never come across it. We only encounter atomic matter and have built our chemistry around it. So chemistry, like much of science, has huge gaps in it). In this book I point out some of the desperate gaps in modern science. My basic one is incontestable, and I simply explore it as a huge anomaly. Why are we conscious? Consciousness is the only thing we are directly aware of; yet there is no theory of it. Modern

Why Are We Conscious? A Scientist's Take on Consciousness and Extrasensory Perception
David E. H. Jones

ISBN 978-981-4774-32-1 (Hardcover), 978-1-315-16688-9 (eBook)
www.panstanford.com

biochemistry claims that we are all made entirely of atoms. Nothing made of atoms should be conscious: but we are. Nobody understands how a brain can be conscious. Attempts to make a conscious computer have so far not been successful. I extend the puzzle of consciousness by invoking one of the most important hypothesis of the 1900s: the unconscious mind. It is a common psychiatric assumption that we all have one. Indeed, psychiatrists often claim to have recovered some memory or personal characteristic that has been 'repressed' into it. Nobody has any way of exploring it—introspection, of course, simply allows you to scan your conscious mind. The contents and size of the unconscious mind are simply not known. One biological theory is that the higher animals have unconscious minds as well. Since they seem to be conscious too, I tie these ideas together. I make the bold claim that in order to be conscious at all, you need an unconscious mind. This does not explain consciousness, that strange property of a few specialized systems of atoms, but it fits smoothly into evolution theory. Evolution does away with sharp transitions, which may have contributed to its opposition by theology. Theology requires a sharp transition: an animal ape has offspring which are human. By contrast, evolution supposes that certain apes evolved smoothly into mankind. Given that they already had unconscious minds, and were already conscious, the evolutionary process merely requires that (among other changes) their brains, voice boxes and hands greatly improved their functioning.

My notion that there is an unknown world outside the diving bell of our physical space, and that the unconscious mind can sometimes make contact with it, is much more contentious. Indeed, it is entirely possible simply to deny that there is any unknown world out there at all. And yet, such rare human abilities as telepathy, the ability to guess a little better than chance, and to induce seemingly non-material acoustic 'raps' (I give many details in Chapters 8 to 11) seem to support the existence of such a world. Humans make contact with that world very rarely and irreproducibly. I explore the notion that such contact, where it occurs, does so via the unconscious mind. That idea fits two powerful examples in which humans have obtained useful information from that world. Chapter 15 gives details of Myers's 'cross-correspondences' and Bond and Alleyne's discoveries about the Edgar Chapel at Glastonbury. Both involved the transfer of information by 'automatic writing', which seems to be a way of activating the unconscious mind, and both seemed to imply that the world outside our diving bell contains once-human entities with information. An interesting counter-example, which seemed not to invoke any once-human entities in that world, was created in the 1970s by the Toronto Society for Psychical Research (Chapters 6 and 11 have many details). That Society invented the entirely fictional ghost Philip. A group of eight people, none claiming any 'psychic' ability, made up Philip's history and character and obtained clear physical phenomena—rapping noises and table movements. They did not, however, obtain any information from Philip which had not been devised beforehand by the members of the group. Their experiment seemed not to look for information unknown to any human mind, but present in the unknown world. I suspect, however, that such information is copiously there.

At present, the unknown world cannot be detected by anything other than by the unconscious human mind. Even that contact is (in my view) both occasional and deceptive. Alan Turing in his famous paper 'Can a Machine Think?'[35] mentions the human skill of telepathy, which cannot be duplicated by a machine and which (Chapter 8) I ascribe to the unconscious mind. I regard the properties and even the existence of the unknown world as a tentative personal notion of my own—although in Chapter 12 I note that many non-scientists seem to believe in something similar. I propose in Chapter 16 that advances in artificial intelligence might provide positive technical evidence, but this would require a new development. It would mean the making of a computer with an unconscious mind, and I have no idea how it might be done. Another physical test which I suggest is based on my calculation in Chapter 7 that the unknown world is extremely cold. It may be at about 10 K compared to the 290 K or so of our earthly world. If there is even a weak coupling between the two worlds, any material object should cool down very slowly if deprived of thermal energy from the physical world.

Meanwhile, this book amasses and looks critically at many of the claims of 'parapsychology', which seems to be largely concerned with the doings of the unconscious mind. I have tried to study such claims from a scientific perspective, as Henry Sidgwick and his followers aimed to do in the Psychical Research Society from 1882 onwards (Chapter 14). Many parapsychological findings seem not to be scientifically credible: but as James Carpenter remarked, 'Parapsychologists must deal in preposterous propositions anyway.'[7] In the course of my study I have encountered many dubious claims and have tried to maintain a fair balance between baffled acceptance and scientific scepticism. Many times I have been tempted to soften or dilute my statements so as to increase my chances of being right. As Irving Good once remarked, 'The art of being correct lies in making the weakest possible statements.' Nonetheless, I have tried to resist this steady temptation to hedge my bets. Any of my conclusions may just be wrong, and quickly disprovable.

My feeling (and it is just a feeling) remains that the physical world of atoms in space is not the only one—

although it is the only one currently accessible to scientific instruments. Outside our diving bell there may indeed be some unknown world. I echo a famous remark by the physicist Niels Bohr: 'Your theory is crazy; the question is whether it's crazy enough to be true.'

Appendix A

A Brief Account of Some of the Laws of Chance: Practical Applications of Statistics

THE LAWS OF CHANCE WERE first worked out in the 1700s by mathematicians. They soon adopted the useful convention that an absolute impossibility has a chance value of 0 and an absolute certainty a value of 1. (The chance of an unbiased coin coming down 'heads' is thus exactly 0.5.) They were soon able to deduce, for example, the overall probability that if two chancy events are set up together neither, either or both will happen. Their theory rapidly came to dominate quite complicated games of chance, such as whist. Gradually probabilistic thinking came to dominate science more generally, and then practical sociology, especially on a large scale. Indeed the word *statistical* comes from linguistic roots meaning 'state arithmetic'.

The tradition of modern scientific publication is that the author only presents significant findings. Thus if a scientific paper gives a number such as 3.1 units, it means anything between 3.05 and 3.14 units. The calculations behind that number might have been made to many places of decimals, but the author only give the result to the precision that the experiment or observation seemed to imply. These days, numbers are often given as (say) 3.1 ± 0.05, implying sort of defined limit. An alternative, and usually a bit of shrewd guesswork, is to imply a Gaussian distribution (I define this below). Thus 3.1 (0.05) might imply a Gaussian distribution whose central point is 3.1, and whose standard deviation around that point is 0.05.

Many sciences have their own conventions about statistical accuracy. I recall, for example, learning the limits of chemical analysis. You had to find the proportion of each element in your compound to within 0.3 percent. If several analyses failed to achieve this, you were forced to publish (for example) 'nitrogen consistently low'. Chemical readers might understand your problem. Otherwise, they would simply take your compound as impure, and disregard any properties you wanted to report for it.

This steady advance of probability and statistics into experimental work did not go unchallenged. The eminent physicist Lord Rutherford once said, 'If your experiment needs statistics, you ought to have done a better experiment.' Rutherford's denunciation was probably aimed at experiments with such large errors that their perpetrators needed to scratch around by statistical methods to reach any conclusion at all. The ideal experiment (like many of those published by Rutherford himself) would have such a stunning and definitive outcome that you would never need to worry about small errors. Few of us are Rutherfords, however. Most of us have to be very familiar with experimental errors—how to minimize them wherever possible, and how to handle them statistically when they still intrude. Often they are simply annoying. An accurate chemical analysis, for example, might prove a point unambiguously; a vague one leaves two or more possibilities open, and the chemist has to resolve the puzzle by some separate investigation. Sometimes, however, experimental or observational errors dominate a study entirely. Parapsychology is often like this.

The limit we are most interested in here is 'noise'. It is universal and occurs whenever a technique is pushed to its limits. Thus if you turn up a sonic amplifier, you will hear the random movement of the electrons in its input stages as a rushing noise. If you try to measure a microgram on a balance designed to respond to 10 micrograms, you will find that the display wanders randomly and fails to indicate a clear number. The 'paranormal' experiments I discuss are usually dominated by noise to such an extent that it takes clever statistical analysis of the results to show that any effect has been revealed at all.

One obvious way to clarify this state of affairs is simply to do the whole experiment again. Many experiments (such as those to discover if a new drug has a useful medical effect) are almost meaningless unless conducted a large number of times. At some stage, however, it makes sense to stop and look at the findings so far. Rather than ploughing ahead with still more experimental work, it is easier to apply mathematical statistics to what you have got so far. The usual trick is to set up a 'null hypothesis', that the results mean nothing and are due to pure noise or pure chance, and then use statistical mathematics to try and find out how likely this would be. A result 'significant at the 0.1 level', for example, might have arisen by chance once in ten times. Many scientists denounce this criterion as unconvincing. They argue for a smaller number such as 0.01 (which implies that the results might have arisen by chance only once in 100 times).

If (as is the fate of many paranormalists) you do lots of ambiguous experiments, you are likely to wind up with a mass of results which show between them a lot of noise and scatter. Experimentalists are always on the lookout for patterns of scatter which fit specific sorts of 'distribution'. With good luck a pattern will suggest a known distribution that instantly suggests what has been going on. Furthermore, many statistical results have already been worked out for every known distribution. You can look up the appropriate one and apply it at once. The Poisson distribution and the Gaussian distribution are particularly well known and useful. The Gaussian distribution, the famous 'bell-shaped curve' named for the great mathematician Karl Gauss, is commonly assumed in many findings. Suppose, for example, you toss an unbiased coin many times and record for each trial the number of 'heads' against the total number of tosses. When you plot the results on graph paper, you will find a close approximation to a Gaussian distribution. It will peak at about 0.5, but the bell-shaped curve will also reflect many results close to this. The 'standard deviation' of the Gaussian curve (roughly, how wide it is) shows how closely the results cluster about the most likely value. The extreme rims of the bell show the occasional improbability. They reveal the few occasions on which by pure chance the coin has fallen 'heads' much more often that you would expect, or much less often.

Practical applications of statistics

The commonest example of statistics is probably the 'poll' by which sociologists try to work out what a nationwide survey would reveal. Polls of a few thousand people can often decide (with a small but calculable likely error) what a whole-nation survey, such as an election, would discover. There are lots of opportunities for mistakes. Thus a poll based on a telephone survey only includes those who own telephones—an error which has caused trouble in the past. And some social problems are beyond any useful poll. Hence, for example, Lord Leverhulme's mournful dictum 'Half the money I spend on advertising is wasted. But I don't know which half!'

Appendix B

Some Statistical Calculations about Those 'Star Guessers' Who Can Often Guess Cards a Bit Better Than Chance

HERE I TRY TO MAKE some estimates of the guessing power of some 'star guessers', using the few reports of card-guessing games which give the actual numbers of correct and incorrect guesses. Most publications usually just say that the results were very unlikely to arise by chance, but a few publications give enough data for me to calculate how well the star guesser actually did. My mathematical approach divides the guesses into two. One set of findings is correct by consisting of correct psychic predictions; the other set is made up of random guesses whose success or failure is due to pure chance. Their sum gives the total predictive power of the guesser.

In a 1930s test of the then new Zener cards, the experimenter Rhine tried them on the star guesser Adam Linzmayer. Linzmayer guessed 1500 cards and got 404 of them correct. Since a Zener card has a 0.2 chance of being chosen correctly by chance, a purely chance score would have been 0.2 times 1500, i.e. 300. Let us imagine that Linzmayer had a psychic predictive accuracy of 8.7 percent. In my terminology that means of his guesses, 8.7 percent were inspired and totally correct, while 91.3 percent were merely random. Out of 1500 trials, therefore, he would score $1500 \times 0.087 = 130$ correct psychic guesses, plus $1500 \times 0.913 \times 0.2 = 274$ correct random guesses, a total of 404 correct guesses—which is what he did actually score.

In another set of card-guessing experiments, Rhine worked with the remarkable guesser Hubert Pearce. Out of 1850 trials, Pearce scored 558 correct guesses when 370 (again, 1 in 5) would have been expected by chance. This gives him an excess over chance of 12.7 percent.

These figures are not untypical. Another case with useful numbers is Samuel Soal's publication of 1943 about the star guesser Basil Shackleton, again on cards of which one was correct out of 5. Out of 3789 guesses that Shackleton made, he got 1083 right, not the 758 that would have occurred by pure chance. His psychic predictive accuracy was thus 10.7 percent. Thirty-five years later, in 1978, Betty Marwick of the Society for Psychical Research conducted a tricky study of the numbers that Soal had used in his randomizations. She concluded that he had retrospectively altered his results and that the true findings were not far from chance. Attempts to replicate them have not succeeded, but the achievements of star guessers can seldom be replicated anyway. The results may be suspect, but I still include them. I do not have much numerical information, and like the idea of trying my calculation on whatever I can find.

Another instance in which my information is suspect or incomplete concerns one of Rhine's experiments of the 1930s on the rolling of dice (I discuss such experiments in Chapter 9). An early experiment using commercial dice gave a score of 3110, when the one predicted for chance guessing would have been would have been 2810. This was later claimed as having only 1 chance in a billion of occurring randomly. My calculation gives it an edge of a mere 4.3 percent over chance, which is perhaps within the expected range for commercial dice.

Records published by Schmidt[32] reveal that his star guesser 'DW' once made 7600 trials, each of which had 1 chance of success in 4, so that a chance-bound expectation would be a quarter of 7600, which is 1900. 'DW' scored 2065. A psychic predictive accuracy of a mere 2.9 percent above chance would have achieved this score. Again, Schmidt tried an experiment with 3 subjects who collectively scored '4.4 percent above chance'. The experiment used 63,000 trials, again with each having a 0.25 chance of being right at random. Accordingly, one might expect 15,750 hits by chance alone. Schmidt recorded 4.4 percent more than this, i.e. 29.4 percent or 18,522 hits. If his team had shown psychic predictive accuracy of 5.9 percent, then you'd expect 3717 psychic hits plus 14,820 chance ones = 18,537, pretty much as observed. Another experiment of Schmidt's used just one subject, 'JB'. A graph of 5000 trials showed some 1365 successes where 1250 might have been expected by chance alone. JB would have needed just 3.1 percent of psychic predictive accuracy to achieve this.

These calculations show that a star guesser does indeed exceed chance, but quite modestly. On average, perhaps, such a guesser has a bit more than a 7 percent edge over a normal chance-bound individual. Schmidt originally used as 'uncaused events' the quantally uncaused nuclear decays of Strontium-90, but later moved to more amenable quantally uncaused events. His results suggest that a star guesser can sometimes acquire information which in quantum theory should not exist. Tests with tables of random numbers seem to show that star guessers can guess these too, but again their guessing skill is only modestly better than chance.

Appendix C

Physics, the Rise of Quantum Mechanics and Decline of Determinism

IN PHYSICS, THE OBSERVABLE UNIVERSE is made up ultimately of fundamental particles. In bulk, they behave in a very predictable Newtonian way. A mass of them, such as a billiard ball, is a particle and not a wave. It can be given any velocity in any direction and can be affected by four fundamental forces. For a billiard ball, mechanical impact applied by a cue is the important one; it comes ultimately from the electromagnetic force released by chemistry in the player's arm. Gravity, which holds the ball on the table, is also important. The ball in fact feels all four physical forces. These are the strong and weak nuclear forces, which hold atomic nuclei together, and these stabilize the atoms of the ball, the electromagnetic force which holds the ball in shape and transmits impacts to it, and gravity, which is an outsider. Billiards, being a branch of physics, is rational and predicable–so that a player of billiards hones his physical skill and does not blame chance if he loses to a more skilful one. Indeed, the many successful predictions of Newtonian physics (e.g. those of eclipses) helped the Victorian belief that physics was essentially already perfect and complete. Among its implications was the notion of 'determinism', that the future was determined entirely by the present and by the physical laws which acted on it. In the early 1800s Pierre Laplace, a theoretician who greatly extended Newtonian mechanics, imagined that an intellect which could comprehend all the entities and forces of nature, and was powerful enough to analyse their interactions, would know the whole future. This deterministic philosophy even permeated into the arts. James Thomson, in his depressing poem 'The City of Dreadful Night' (1874) made a character say, 'I find no hint throughout the Universe / Of good or ill, of blessing or of curse; / I find alone Necessity Supreme.' The great Max Planck almost decided not to enter physics at all, as there was so little of importance still left to do!

However, Planck did enter physics, and transformed it. About 1900 his first revolutionary claim was that light was both a particle and a wave. It came in specific packets dubbed 'photons'. These travelled as particles, but still had a frequency and a wavelength. On the human scale, of course (as in calculations for lenses), we take the simple Newtonian view that light is merely a set of particles travelling at a certain speed.

Photons were found to obey a very strange form of physics: 'quantum mechanics'. Within a few decades, all the basic physical entities had been 'quantized'. One of the simpler rules of quantum mechanics is that of discontinuity. A billiard ball can have any energy and any speed. In the quantum world, only specific values are possible. Thus an electron in an atom can have a few allowed amounts of energy, but never anything intermediate. A nucleus can have one of a few finite levels of spin, but again, nothing intermediate. In the ordinary world, an object is either a particle or a wave (a billiard ball is a particle in that world); in the quantum world, it is both. One might even be able to predict the behaviour of a billiard ball by taking it as a wave with a very short wavelength—though the largest particle whose wave character has been studied is a clump of 60 atoms. (There are over 10^{22} atoms in a billiard ball.)

Even more strange is the principle of indeterminacy, as proposed in 1925 by Werner Heisenberg. He said that there was a limit on submicroscopic exactitude. If you examine an electron, for example, the more you know about its position, the less you know about its velocity. This is not just a limitation of physical technique. An electron does not have an exact position and velocity, only a combination of the two. The coupling of the pair comes out of the theory. The velocity of an electron, for example, has no precise value, only a probability: and probabilities these days get everywhere in physics. Thus the feeble reflection of light at a glass interface, which had puzzled Newton, is now ascribed to probability. A photon has a 4 percent chance of being reflected at a glass surface, and a 96 percent chance of being transmitted. No physicist can say any more than that.

Thus modern fundamental physics has abandoned determinism in favour of chance. Some atomic nuclei, for example, are radioactive: they are unstable and will sooner or later eject a particle or even fission into two others. You can never predict such a decay. The best you can do is to construct a 'half-life' such that half the nuclei of a sample will have decayed in that time. Decay itself, says quantum mechanics, is an 'uncaused event'. Both the complete nucleus and its decay products continue in some odd way to exist, as a superposition of 'state vectors'. Only when an observer looks at the nucleus or its decay products do those vectors 'collapse' into one specific state.

In 1928 the cosmologist Arthur Eddington claimed that the unintelligibility of quantum mechanics was a virtue. He said that laws we understand are not laws at all, but conventions erected by our minds to satisfy themselves. The laws of quantum mechanics are the first real laws to be discovered and may be recognized as such by the very fact that they do not satisfy the mind's craving for intelligibility. Quantum mechanics seems to claim not only that we can never determine the exact properties of a microsystem, but that it hasn't got any. Various interpretations of the puzzle have been built–that of the great Scandinavian physicist Niels Bohr is known as 'the Copenhagen interpretation'. The fact remains that quantum mechanics, the current basic physics of the smallest systems, gives correct predictions but, unlike classical physics, does not reduce to a set of intelligible common-sense principles. All science is fundamentally physics (the mighty physicist Lord Rutherford once said, 'Science can be divided into two branches: physics and stamp-collecting'), so the current state of scientific theory seems very unsatisfactory. All existing science is ultimately built on quantum mechanics.

Fortunately, its weirdness 'averages away' to normal predictable Newtonian behaviour on almost every technical scale. Technology continues to go from strength to strength. Buildings and bridges stand up as before, engines are successfully designed to run, and chemicals to work. But the theory beneath them has changed completely. Despite its seeming denial of common sense, quantum mechanics flourishes, and indeed has extended its stranglehold. The Russian politician Beria once asked the physicist Kurchatov if the principles of quantum mechanics conflicted with Marxism-Leninism. He got the reply, 'I don't know, Comrade. But you can't have the Bomb without them.'

Hugh Everett III and his proposal for explaining quantum mechanics

A clever solution to some of the puzzles of quantum mechanics was suggested by Hugh Everett III in 1957. It featured lots of unobservable universes. Everett proposed that whenever a quantum choice arose, the whole universe split into two–in one of which it occurred, and in the other of which it did not. Our own universe is the outcome of billions of quantum choices which are now historical–they happened or they did not happen. Everett felt that there should also be billions of other universes whose quantized choices had been different.

This theory seems rather similar to the notions I am putting forward in this book. Indeed, it makes me seem almost modest. I am proposing just one extra world, of which we can even get an occasional glimpse: Everett has postulated vast numbers of unobservable universes. But his bold theory has several problems. One is simple–where are all these unobservable universes? If space is indeed infinite, it has lots of room for them. And just one extra dimension of space (I discuss dimensions in Chapter 7) would give even more. Even so, Everett's theory has not been widely adopted. The physicist John Bell (he of Bell's inequality) said of it, 'If you take it seriously, it is hard to take anything else seriously.' Another problem is that it seems to dodge what is in quantum mechanics a basic item of information–the probability of an 'uncaused event'. If you can never determine anything, you should at least be able to calculate a precise probability, which Everett's theory seems not to do.

Schrödinger's cat in quantum mechanics

Erwin Schrödinger was one of the founders of quantum mechanics but always had reservations about it. He is claimed once to have said of it, 'I don't like it, and I'm sorry I ever had anything to do with it.' His famous paradox of 1935 reminds me of the more recent quantum experiments of Alain Aspect. In these, a nuclear decay releases two photons that travel off not merely in opposite directions, but with perpendicular polarizations. Quantum theory alleges that the two photons by themselves do not have any axis of polarization; only the pair has that property. These polarization axes are, however, mutually perpendicular. Once you have determined the polarization axis of one photon, the axis of the other has to be perpendicular to it. Aspect indeed found that when you had determined the polarization axis of one photon, the other was found to have a perpendicular one—even though they were by then so far apart that no information could be transmitted from one to the other. They remained in some way 'quantally entangled'. Schrödinger claimed in his paradox that a cat could be entangled with a single radioactive nucleus. He imagined his cat shut in a box with a mechanism by which a lethal dose of hydrogen cyanide gas would be released by the 'uncaused' quantum decay of one nucleus in the mechanism. A cat is a macroscopic creature, and its properties (which will be described by some horrendously complicated quantum-mechanical wave function) will be vastly different if is dead than if it is alive. Even so, it would neither be alive nor dead until an observer opened the box and looked in to resolve the entanglement. A machine looking it (such as a camera) would not resolve the paradox: it would merely adopt a superposed vector state too. Only a conscious observer could 'collapse the wave function' and see the cat as alive or dead. I have pondered that this might in some way link quantum mechanics usefully with consciousness. (Roger Penrose and Stuart Hameroff have proposed a subtle link between the two based on the microtubules that occur in brain neurons.) I myself cannot see any useful connection between quantum mechanics and consciousness, but both may be relevant to that weak coupling I postulate between the physical and the unknown world.

For the moment, however, I am content to propose a challenge for Hugh Everett III. In Schrödinger's cat experiment, choose a system which has only a 1 percent chance of decay. The cat then has only a 1 percent chance of dying. Does the universe split into 100 new ones, in 99 of which the cat is alive, and in 1 of which it is dead? And suppose you make the probability an 'irrational fraction' like $1/\pi$? Such an irrational fraction can never be represented by a whole-number ratio x/y such that the cat lives in x universes but dies in y of them.

I used to reckon that Schrödinger's paradox, with its 'uncaused nuclear decay', could be powerfully tested by seeing if a star guesser could guess a decay a little better than chance. If he or she could not, it would indeed be truly 'uncaused', as quantum mechanics asserts. Helmut Schmidt[32] has done the test (Appendix B) and has found that star guessers can predict radioactive decays slightly better than by pure chance. This reinforces my feeling that a star guesser somehow accesses information outside our diving bell.

The decline of determinism. The scientific picture of the physical world had two ambitions: (a) to make correct predictions and (b) to make sense. 'Classical' science—Newtonian physics, Daltonian chemistry, Darwinian biology—did both. The most basic principle of modern physics, that of the quantum theory, only seems to manage (a). It does not make sense, and it denies an important principle of classical physics, determinism.

Determinism made the apparent freedom of the human and animal 'will' very puzzling. Eddington once speculated that human 'free will' is real and exists because the brain somehow amplifies quantum mechanical uncertainty up into the observable world. Conversely, that freedom was wittily denied in a limerick by Maurice Hare: 'There once was a man who said Damn! / It is borne in upon me I am / An engine that moves in predestinate grooves, / I'm not even a bus, I'm a tram.' If we are indeed not buses but trams, human beings and animals generally are merely complicated but basically deterministic robots. Even so, free will would have powerful advantages. If evolution could create it, it would augment any living organism. At the very least, if your behavior were free and unpredictable, predators would not be able to predict it. (This may explain why it is so hard to catch a fly.)

Einstein did not like this retreat from determinism at all. 'Der Herrgott würfelt nicht' (God does not play dice), he said. I share Einstein's discomfort at admitting 'uncaused' quantum-mechanical events into physics. I myself reckon that human free will arises from ordinary biological sloppiness (Chapter 3), but I agree with Eddington that there is something to be explained.

Another assault on determinism was mounted in about the 1960s and grew with the development of the computer. This was chaos theory. If you know the state of a mechanism exactly at one time, you can use the deterministic laws to compute its state at any future time. Unfortunately, your initial conditions always have a slight error. In a chaotic system, that error builds up very fast. Any prediction for the distant future is then pretty much worthless. This is the sort of accumulating error which makes it impossible to forecast the weather for more than a few days ahead. I have a clever battery-operated toy which exploits chaos theory; you cannot guess whether any rotating element will turn clockwise or anticlockwise, or when or how it will change direction. Chaos theory puts limits on the number and character of the various forms of chaos.

This abandonment of determinism does not imply that the future is undetermined. It merely means that you cannot determine it from the present. The future a year hence, or a million years hence for that matter, may be already exactly certain. John Calvin's religious predestination notion, that when a child is born it is already certain whether its soul will go to hell, may be quite correct. A view of the future (though nobody can derive it from the present) shows the soul of that child in hell. The idea that you can predict the future from the present works in many cases, but Laplace's idealistic notion that it should work universally is just that—an idealistic notion.

Appendix D

The Brain as an Information Store, and Information Outside It

My overall sense is that the brain is not primarily a memory store. Many of the memories which it retains appear to be held in, or at least accessed through, a small region of it called the hippocampus. Both in human beings and in animals, the main function of the brain seems to be controlling the body; it is chiefly a body administrator. Human beings seem to owe their great intellectual power largely to a uniquely high brain weight compared to the weight of the body. A big brain may have enough unused capacity to think about what it is doing, and to remember what it has done. So it is worthwhile trying to guess its informational storage capacity.

I have proposed, not very seriously, that like many computers, it uses the same microstructure for both memory and processing. In the course of life it fills up with memory, so that the space it has for data processing gets steadily reduced. Ultimately, malfunctions occur: this is senility. When the brain is finally full up, we die.[17] This hypothesis implies that being stupid, ignorant or forgetful helps to keep the brain empty and is a recipe for long life.

I have also calculated that, purely as an identifier, we all have to carry at least 33 bits of information outside the brain.[16] It is worth looking into the matter more seriously.

Nobody knows how the brain holds information. Many technological schemes for holding information need moving parts (such as a rotating disc, for example), but the brain has no moving parts. One theory is that it holds data as recirculating pulses (an early computer memory held information this way). This theory requires a few neurons connected in a small loop, each triggering the next. A stored bit of information goes round and round the loop as a recirculating pulse. Another theory is that a neuron stores information by its content of 'neurotransmitter' chemical substances. Each neurotransmitter activates a special 'receptor' inside the neuron and this receptor accumulates. It accumulates. When it exceeds some critical value, the neuron fires and depletes it. Lots of neurotransmitters are known: they include acetylcholine, adrenaline, norepinephrine, serotonin, histamine, dopamine, and gamma-amino butyric acid.

These two theories, recirculating pulses or stored neurotransmitters, seem to be the main ideas about how the brain holds information. If anyone ever constructed electronic equivalents, the obvious thing would be to make lots of them, connect them together in various ways, and discover if the assembly ever behaved anything like a brain. In particular, the investigators should try to make it remember something.

What limit might these theories place on the amount of information in a brain? A typical human brain has about one hundred billion (10^{11}) neurons. The recirculating-pulse theory suggests that maybe 5 neurons are needed to store 1 bit, so the whole brain (if it were all used just for memory) could hold at most 2×10^{10} bits, or 0.02 terabits. The neurotransmitter theory implies that just one neuron might hold several bits of data, one for each of neurotransmitters it uses. Let us assume that on average it uses 10 of them. An average neuron can then hold 10 bits. A whole brain could then hold 10^{12} bits or 1 terabit. Suppose we take in 1000 bits of nerve data every second, that is about 10^8 bits a day. If we live for 3×10^4 days, that is 3×10^{12} bits of sensory input. That is 3 terabits.

This calculation is unavoidably a very rough estimate of the data storage capacity of the human brain, but already it suggests that each of us may know more than our brain can hold. Of course, the brain may store much more than this. On the other hand, if most of it is a mere body administrator with little space to hold information, and sometimes duplicates what it does hold, it may hold less. My sense is that the brain is mainly administrative, and only a small about of it handles our memories. Our conscious memory can probably not bring up anything like a terabit of information; much of our knowledge must take the form of physical skills (such being able to breathe, or walk, or use a hammer) that we know, but do not think of as held in the memory. And, of course, much important data may be stored in the unconscious mind, about which we know essentially nothing. The novelist William Gerhardie felt that the unconscious mind greatly exceeds the conscious one. He likened human beings to icebergs, of which only a small proportion appears above the surface. I like the comparison, but since we know nothing about the size of the unconscious mind, we cannot guess how much information it may need to store, whether inside or outside the brain. Furthermore, the brain may not be not intensively used. Not only does it seem constantly ready to grab new experiences and place them in memory; it seems to hold back-up copies of important knowledge. Thus if information is lost, there is a good chance that it can be found elsewhere in the brain. The victim of a stroke (I discuss the matter in my discussion of strokes in Chapter 3) may slowly recover seemingly lost memories or abilities.

The space that the brain needs for its information could, of course, be greatly reduced by cunning coding. Computers code information routinely, but I have argued, also in Chapter 3, that the brain seems not to go in for coding.

Others besides myself have pondered the way we may hold our memories and skills. The great biologist J. B. S. Haldane disliked the notion that if someone made a perfect, atom-for-atom copy of his own brain, the result would have all his memories. Marilyn Monroe was notorious among film directors for forgetting her lines. She once claimed that her memory was so limited that she could not remember a new telephone number without forgetting an old one. The poet Oliver Goldsmith once saluted a classics scholar: '. . . and still the wonder grew / That one small head could carry all he knew.' Even so, I suspect that the brain does not hold information in the precise way that a computer holds it. Precision of any kind would be completely out of place in a biological object like a brain.

Several science fiction stories have imagined the contents of a human brain getting transferred to another human brain. Sometimes this process transfers the 'identity' of the donor as well: he or she gets to see with the eyes of the recipient and acquires a whole lot of new memories amounting to an added life story. This fits in with my feeling that the brain is not intensively used and has room for much new information. I have even read stories in which the contents of a human brain are transferred to a computer memory. However, even in fiction no author seems to have imagined how much information might have to be transferred, or whether the brain holds all the information we know. In its strong form, the discipline of artificial intelligence proposes that any sufficiently complex computer might be conscious. I disagree, but discuss conscious computers in Chapter 16.

My guess here about brain information is at least consistent with the notion that we may hold some information outside the brain: 'in the cloud', so to speak, the cloud being that unknown world. In his novel[8] of 1968. *2001: A Space Odyssey*, Arthur C. Clarke imagined aliens who 'had learnt to store knowledge in the structure of space itself, and to preserve their thoughts for eternity in frozen lattices of light', thus freeing themselves from 'the tyranny of matter'.[8] This is not quite storing information in non-material form 'in the cloud', but it is a big step on the way. I like the idea; it reflects my musings that the human brain may have some sort of ability to acquire and store information in the unknown world outside our diving bell.

Appendix E

The Anthropic Principle

THE ANTHROPIC PRINCIPLE ESSENTIALLY ASSERTS that the universe exists to make conscious intelligent life possible. I present here a rough calculation about it. Let us assume that only the occasional planetary surface can be the abode of life. I will take our Earth as an archetypal planet sustaining life. It has a surface area of 5×10^8 km^2. We expect life to occur in a volume bounded by that surface and perhaps 20 km of oxygenated height (allowing for life in the sea). That makes 10^{10} km^3 of livable volume on the planet Earth. The Earth is a single planet of a single star. If there are 10^{11} stars in a galaxy, 10^{11} observable galaxies, and 10 percent of stars maintain a planet on which life is possible (a wild guess; there may be far fewer), then the total volume of the physical universe which can sustain life is at most 10^{31} km^3. This is a minute fraction, 10^{-39}, of the total available volume. Most life (e.g. plants and bacteria) is not even conscious, let alone intelligent, so intelligent life must be a tiny fraction even of this. Setting it up wastes a lot of time, too: maybe 13 billion years. Life itself started about 3 billion years ago, and intelligent human life perhaps a few million years ago. I deduce that applied to our three-dimensional world, the Anthropic Principle is extremely uneconomic. Might it be a better fit to a universe of more dimensions? I have read that the more dimensions a space has, the more 'nearest neighbours' a point can have, and the more complex the structures that can be made within it. Life itself is very complex, intelligent life even more so. Thus a zero-dimensional space is a featureless point. A one-dimensional frieze can exist in up to seven types; a two-dimensional area (such as a wallpaper) can have 17 different types of symmetric pattern; a three-dimensional volume can have 230 space-groups. The dimensions of our space seem locally to be three of space plus of time, but we do not know the dimensionality of the universe as a whole. (I have discussed dimensionality in Chapter 7; string theorists have postulated up to 11 dimensions for our space.) Yet even an 11-dimensional universe, with perhaps 10^7 nearest neighbours possible for any point in it, would not make the Anthropic Principle convincing. An alternative notion is that intellectual power resides mainly in the unknown world and is transmitted by the unconscious mind to the conscious mind of a human being. This both fits the few facts we have, and seems vaguely compatible with the views I am exploring here.

References

1. Alexander, E., *Proof of Heaven: A Neurosurgeon's Journey into the Afterlife* (Simon and Schuster, 2012).
2. Anderson, J. L., and Spangler, G. W., *Journal of Physical Chemistry* 77 (1973): 3114.
3. Bauby, J.-D., *The Diving Bell and the Butterfly*. This book was first published in French in 1997; an English translation was published by the Knopf Doubleday Publishing Group in 1998.
4. Blegvad, P., *The Book of Leviathan* (Sort Of Books, 2000), Part XI.
5. Bond, F. P., *Gate of Remembrance* (Blackwell, 1918).
6. Brookes-Smith, C., *Journal of the Society for Psychical Research* 47, no. 756 (1973): 69.
7. Carpenter, J., in *Handbook of Parapsychology*, ed. B. B. Wolman (Reinhold 1977), 202, 217.
8. Clarke, A. C., *2001: A Space Odyssey* (Hutchinson, 1968).
9. Crawford, W. J., *The Reality of Psychic Phenomena* (Watkins, 1918).
10. Davenas, E., et al., *Nature* 333 (1988): 816.
11. Dennett, D., and Hofstadter, D., *The Minds's I* (Basic Books, 1981).
12. Derjaguin, B. V., *Scientific American* 223 Nov. (1970): 52.
13. French, A. P., *Newtonian Mechanics* (Thomas Nelson, 1965), 111, 724.
14. Grof, S., *Realms of the Human Unconscious* (Souvenir Press, 1975).
15. Gurney, E., Myers, F. W. H., and Podmore, F., *Phantasms of the Living* (1886; reprinted in 2 volumes by Cambridge University Press, 2011).

16. Jones, D. E. H., *The Inventions of Daedalus* (W. H. Freeman, 1982), 50.
17. Ibid., 142.
18. Jones, D. E. H., *Nature* 372 (1994) 226; *The Further Inventions of Daedalus* (Oxford University Press, 1999), 56.
19. Jones, D. E. H., *The Further Inventions of Daedalus* (Oxford University Press, 1999), 153.
20. Jones, D. E. H., *Chemistry World* 5 no. 3 (2008): 80.
21. Jones, D. E. H., *The Aha! Moment* (Johns Hopkins University Press, 2012), 5.
22. Ibid., 9.
23. Ibid., 15.
24. Ibid., 117.
25. Ibid., 234.
26. Libet, B., *Mind Time* (Harvard University Press, 2005).
27. Mayer, E. L., *Extraordinary Knowing* (Bantam Books, 2000).
28. McMullan, J. T., *Journal of the American Society for Psychical Research* 65 (1971): 493.
29. Morrison, P., and Morrison, P., *Powers of Ten* (Scientific American Library/W. H. Freeman, 1982).
30. Owen, I. M., and Sparrow, M. H., *Conjuring Up Philip* (Harper and Row, 1976).
31. Porges, A., *The Devil and Simon Flagg* (Richard Simms Publications, 2009).
32. Schmidt, H., *New Scientist* 44 no. 2 (1969): 114; no. 13 (1971), 757.
33. Shute, N., *No Highway* (Heinemann, 1948).
34. Trivers, R., *Annals of the New York Academy of Science* 207 (2000): 114.
35. Turing, A. M., *Mind* 59 (1950): 433.
36. Wells, H. G., 'Under the Knife', in *The Short Stories of H. G. Wells* (Ernest Benn, 1927), 455.
37. Wolman, B. B. (ed.), *Handbook of Parapsychology* (Reinhold, 1977).
38. Wright, D. A., 'A Theory of Ghosts', *The Worm Runner's Digest* 12 (1971): 95; *A Random Walk in Science*, ed. R. L. Weber (Institute of Physics, 1975), 110.
39. Wyndham, J., *The Chrysalids* (Michael Joseph, 1955).

Index